GREEN JUICES
FOR BEGINNERS

Carla Zaplana

GREEN JUICES FOR BEGINNERS

A ONE-STOP GUIDE TO CLEANSING YOUR BODY

h.f.ullmann

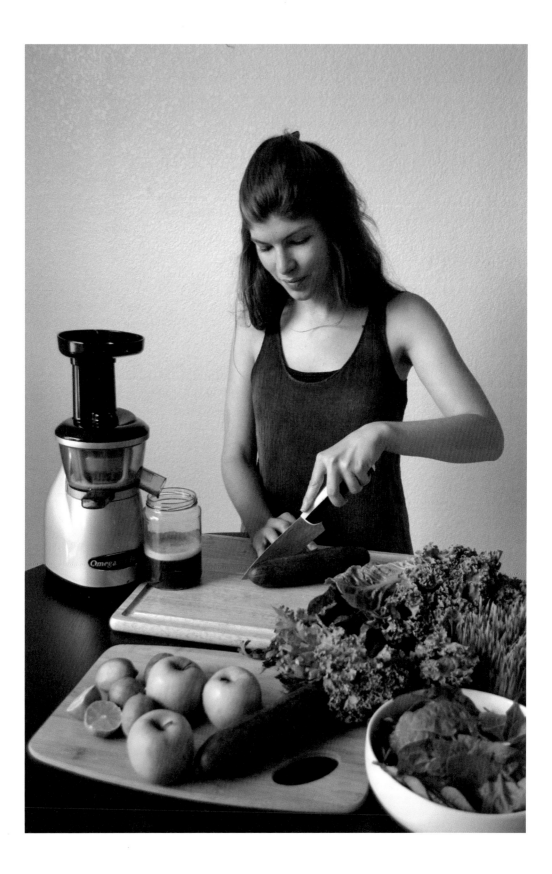

INTRODUCTION

The story of my love affair with green juices is one borne of passion and boundless enthusiasm. I found myself hooked from the very first sip. To this day, I still delight in telling people about the resounding impact green juices have had on my life. There is not a single member of my family who has not, at the very least, given green juices a try, and none of my patients ever leaves a consultation without having been convinced that green juices are the perfect panacea for a healthy life.

I discovered this green elixir at a point in my life when everything seemed off-kilter: I was having to get used to a new country, a new culture, different customs, unfamiliar types of food—all these changes impacted on my physical and emotional state. I put on weight, developed pimples on my face, and, what struck me most, felt devoid of all energy. I no longer felt cheerful; and smiling, which had always been one of my natural characteristics, became a thing of the past.

My unshakable belief in the healing power of certain foods led me to examine the eating habits of my new homeland more carefully and consequently opened my eyes, in particular, to the manipulation and monopolization exercised by the food industry. I therefore decided to alter my own dietary habits and to seek alternative philosophies to all that I had learnt at university. This, in turn, aroused my interest in a diet based on plant products. I began to study the blogs written by experts on vegan diets, such as Dr. Joel Fuhrman, Dr. Neal Barnard, Dr. Mark Hyman, Kris Carr, and Kimberly Snyder. I read numerous books on the subject, one of which, in particular, I recommend time and time again: *China Study*. This book by Dr. T. Colin Campbell argues the case for a vegan diet and is based on scientific studies examining the effects on the human body of a diet based on animal products. I began to realize that not only was my diet starting to change, but my lifestyle as well.

My various ailments were diminishing every day. This encouraged me to alter my diet still further. I got back to my old weight and the pimples on my face disappeared; I no longer felt so exhausted and my spirits lifted again. The high point for me, however, was the discovery of green juices, which I incorporated with great anticipation into my new dietary regime: after all, if merely increasing the intake of vegetable products had produced such positive results and restored me to my true self, what more might I expect if I started the day off with a veritable Molotov cocktail of vegetables? And you know what? There is nothing better! The energy, vitality, and sense of optimism that this drink gave me each morning was almost unbelievable. I completely abandoned coffee, which I had always relied on to get me moving in the past. This green elixir gave me such an energy boost that I remained alert and full of vitality all day long. I began to experiment with different combinations of vegetables. Since I was familiar with the beneficial properties of all the ingredients, I began to experiment with home remedy drinks for all kinds of ailments: headaches, constipation, dizziness, acne, signs of aging, etc.—so much so that my friends began jokingly to call me "Miss Green Juice," a title I found I liked.

Green juices made all my problems disappear: my energy levels rose exponentially, my creativity and enthusiasm blossomed as if a new spring were awakening within me. I believe that the remarkable improvement not only in my physical and mental well-being but also in my emotional state was a direct result of enriching my diet in this extraordinary way. Green juices led me to pay more attention to what I was eating and to eliminate all the toxins in my life. The saying "you are what you eat" is absolutely true, and nowadays I continue to pile my plate high with crudités and eat to keep myself vital, happy, full of optimism, and able to enjoy what I do. This led me to my other passion: raw food.

As I write these words, I almost feel as if I am talking about the first love of my life, as if I am hopelessly besotted by green juices—but that is exactly how it feels, and I do not suppose I shall ever feel any differently. That is why I have ventured to write this, my very first book, as a way of publicizing the positive effects of green juices so that you too may experience for yourself and benefit from their valuable properties. Who knows? Green juices may well end up changing your life too!

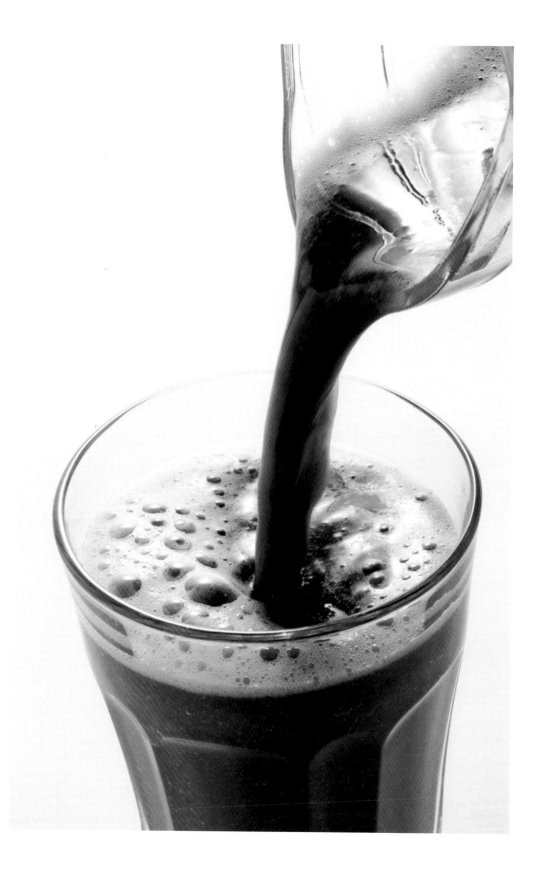

THE POSITIVE EFFECTS OF GREEN JUICES

Making green juices an integral part of our diet can have a very positive effect on our health, as they have outstanding antioxidant, cleansing, and anti-aging properties.

WHAT ARE GREEN JUICES?

Green juices are juices derived from vegetables, primarily leafy greens, such as spinach, lettuce, cress, kale, mustard leaves, rocket, Swiss chard, parsley, etc. The addition of fruit helps make the mixture sweeter.

Green juices are energy bombs as their main constituents are:

Water: more than 65 percent of the human body is water, which is involved in all bodily functions. Green juices provide us with high-quality fluids.

Proteins: green juices supply us with large quantities of amino acids which are very easily absorbed by the body.

Carbohydrates: green juices are full of carbohydrates (simple sugars and starch). Carbohydrates are the body's main source of energy.

Essential fatty acids: only very small amounts of these are present in vegetable juices; they are derived from green leaves.

Micronutrients: green juices are veritable vitamin and mineral bombs. They are extremely rich in water-soluble vitamins such as group B-type vitamins (with the exception of vitamin B12) and also supply us with fat-soluble vitamins, including A and K, as well as carotene (the precursor of vitamin A).

Enzymes: enzymes act as the motor for all chemical reactions within the body. We could not survive for more than three minutes without them. Enzymes are destroyed if food is heated to over 45° C, which is why green juices are an invaluable source of enzymes.

Phytochemical substances: these are what give plants their color, smell, and texture, and protect them from natural enemies. They play a very similar protective role in the human body thanks to their anti-inflammatory and cancer-inhibiting properties and by strengthening the body's immune system.

THE POSITIVE EFFECTS OF GREEN JUICES

WHAT POSITIVE EFFECTS DO THEY HAVE?

The hectic pace of everyday life often means that we pay little attention to looking after our bodies' internal needs. Stress, depression, environmental pollution, the noxious substances which surround us are all factors which can result in our organisms becoming weakened, in dwindling energy levels or susceptibility to illness. In order to combat these damaging influences, our bodies must receive a healthy supply of vitamins, minerals, active enzymes, and other substances which protect our cells and renew cell tissue. Green juices offer one of the best options for ensuring a healthy supply of micronutrients.

They are not an invention of the 21st century, nor are they a passing fad—they are here to stay.

Vitamin and mineral cocktail
How often have we been told that "five a day" is the recommended daily amount of fruit and vegetables needed to cover our micronutrient requirements? Even so, only a few of us manage to eat the required amount of vegetables. By drinking green juices, we derive the beneficial properties in condensed form from all the plant products contained therein. Mention should also be made of the fact that leafy green vegetables are among the most nutritious foods on our planet: in other words, a single green juice a day will provide the entire daily requirement of micronutrients recommended by the American Dietetics Association (ADA).

De-acidification effect
Blood has a natural pH value of 7.35 to 7.45, making it slightly alkaline as a pH of 7 is neutral. According to Dr. Robert Young's work on the pH formula for an optimum acid–alkaline balance: "The pH level of our internal fluids affects every cell in our bodies. The entire metabolic process depends on a balanced internal alkaline environment. A chronically over-acidic pH corrodes body tissue. If left unchecked, it will interrupt all cellular activities and functions, from the beating of your heart to the neural firing of your brain. In summary, over-acidification interferes with life itself." Other recent studies have also shown that cancer cells cannot proliferate in an alkaline environment. Consequently, regular consumption of green juices helps to prevent serious degenerative diseases such as Alzheimer's or cancer.

Vegetables and ripe fruit are the only natural foods which have a distinct alkaline effect on the body, which is why it is so important to include them as an integral part of our daily diet.

Cleansing effect
The diverse composition of substances supplied by green juices is essential for activating a cleansing effect on the body, which will facilitate weight loss. Since the juices also require no digestion, the body can concentrate its energy on detoxifying, regenerating tissue, and generally improving health.

The blood's oxygen uptake
Green plant products contain a great deal of chlorophyll, the pigment which gives plants their green color. The molecular structure of this plant pigment is almost identical to that of hemoglobin—a protein which is responsible for transporting oxygen in the blood to all the cells in the body. This similarity means that chlorophyll thus absorbed is quickly transformed into hemoglobin in the body, thereby increasing the blood's uptake of oxygen. Oxygen is the most important element for keeping cells alive and functioning properly.

Regulating the digestive processes
Although green juice does not contain a great deal of fiber—since the fruit and vegetable pulp and peel are discarded during preparation—it can nevertheless be useful if you suffer from constipation problems. Depending on the type of juicer you use, the juices will still contain at least a certain amount of solid material. This fiber helps stimulate intestinal function.

If you regularly suffer from bloating or irritable bowel syndrome, I recommend that you strain the juice thoroughly before drinking.

Delaying the aging process
Green juices are rich in antioxidants, the main task of which is to combat free radicals—in other words, molecules which damage the body's cells and accelerate the aging process. Free radicals are, of course, formed as a result of natural metabolic processes in organisms, but can also be caused by external factors, such as environmental pollution, tobacco, and industrially manufactured or fried foodstuffs. A healthy lifestyle and an increased consumption of vegetables and green juices are mirrored in strong, shiny hair and softer, healthier, younger skin.

Some green juice fans—myself included—confirm that vegetable juices have helped to reduce the number of wrinkles and fine lines on the face. There is therefore no need for scalpels or chemical-based creams—green juices are your best weapon in the fight against the effects of aging. Always remember that a body which is healthy and beautiful on the inside will be reflected in glowing skin on the outside.

Energy boost

Do you get out of bed each morning filled with a desperate need for a cup of coffee in order to be able to "function" properly? Just try a green juice and you will see how wide awake you suddenly feel. This green elixir is packed with energy and vitality. As mentioned above, it provides us with large quantities of micronutrients, such as vitamins, minerals, and, above all, active enzymes.

As this is in liquid form, the body docs not need to set any digestive processes in motion. In other words, all the nutrients contained in the juice are directly absorbed by the blood, producing a feeling of vitality and an immediate boost of energy that will surprise you.

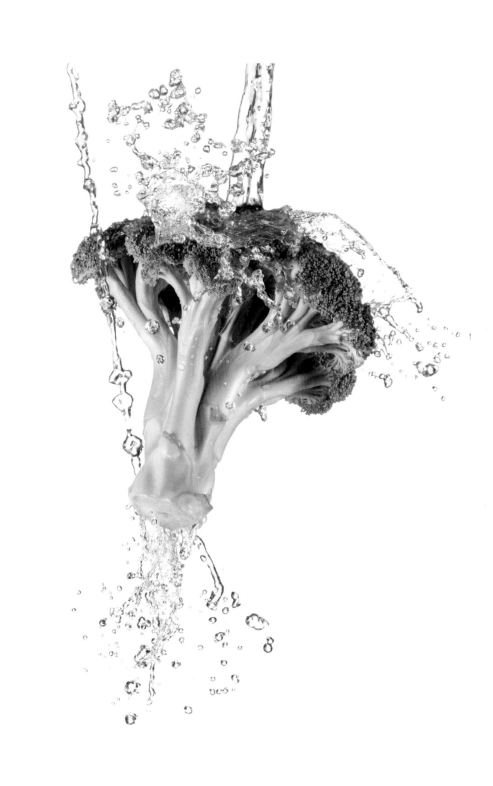

PREPARING GREEN JUICES

The following pages look at which juicer is most suitable for your needs, which is the best magic formula for preparing your own juices and how you can improve the quality of your juices without putting too much strain on your purse.

WHAT EQUIPMENT DO YOU NEED FOR JUICING?

Regardless of whether you have only just discovered the world of green juices or whether they are already part of your daily ritual, at some point you will need an efficient juice extractor.

To this end, I shall continue by discussing some examples of various models currently on the market, comparing their advantages and disadvantages, so that you can decide on the most appropriate model for your own purposes.

Centrifugal juicer

The centrifugal extractor is the most common type of juicer. It has a cylindrical mouth in the center through which to feed in the fruit and vegetables. It opens into a metal basket which acts as a filter. The base of the basket is covered in tiny grater teeth which grate the produce into tiny pieces as the machine spins at high speed. The fast spinning action of the basket crushes the pieces of vegetable against the filter wall, extracting the juice, which is forced out of the flesh and channeled out through a small opening. The pulp, in other words the leftover solid bits, remain inside the juicer and are sent into a separate compartment through another aperture.

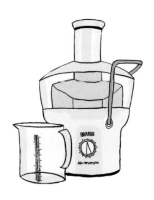

Advantages:
– Fastest way to extract juice. This type of machine extracts the juice directly and is ideal if you are pressed for time.
– The fruit or vegetables do not need to be cut up into small pieces; this reduces preparation time.
– It is a cost-efficient option.

Disadvantages:
– This type of juicer is not very efficient as a lot of juice gets left behind in the pulp. More vegetables are therefore required to produce the same amount of juice as you would using a cold-press juicer.
– Compared to other juicers, this type of juicer does not always juice leafy greens very well. The following tip may help in this respect: simply roll up the green leaves into a compressed ball. This will increase the amount of juice extracted.

- This juicer can only be used to extract juice. Other models possess additional functions (more on this subject later).
- It also tends to be very noisy.
- It operates at high speed. The fast spinning action generates heat which warms the juice, as well as exposing it to increased levels of oxygen so that it oxidizes. The juice loses a significant amount of nutrients, antioxidants, and enzymes during the process.

Cold-press juicer

A cold-press juicer processes the fruit and vegetables by means of a screw- or spiral-type axle. The vegetables are crushed and pressed against the walls of a metal filter, forcing out the juice and separating it from the fibers. This type of juicer sends the juice and the pulp into two separate containers.

Advantages:
- This type of juicer extracts the juice more slowly than a centrifugal juicer, which prevents the juice becoming heated, thus preserving a greater percentage of micronutrients (vitamins, minerals, and enzymes). In addition, not as much air is whisked into the juice, so it is less oxidized and has a greater nutritional value. It is this aspect of juice extraction which has led to the name "cold-press."

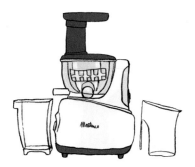

- This type of juicer is suitable for extracting juice from all kinds of fruit and vegetables, including leafy greens and wheat grass.
- The amount of juice extracted is higher and the residual pulp is much drier.
- The machine has various additional functions: for example, it can also produce plant milk and cream from dried fruits, chop up vegetables, and even grind coffee.
- It is quieter than a centrifugal juicer.

Disadvantages:
- It is considerably more expensive.
- The machine takes longer to operate; it works at a lower speed and the chute for adding the ingredients is generally smaller, which is why the vegetables have to be cut up into smaller pieces.

Final considerations before purchasing a juicer

Ideally, when purchasing a juicer, you should be absolutely certain which functions you require and how often you are likely to use it. If you currently have a limited budget and/or are new to the idea of incorporating green juices into your diet, you could save both preparation time and money by purchasing a centrifugal juicer. If you are keen to extract more active substances from your fruit and vegetables and if finances permit, a cold-press juicer is the best option. Not only will it produce more nutrient-rich juice, but it will also save you money on vegetable purchases in the long term. This type of juicer not only extracts more juice from every ingredient but also crushes and processes leafy greens more efficiently. One further factor to be considered is that—as mentioned above—it has more than one function.

Whichever type of juicer you choose, when it comes to cleaning and looking after your machine it is important to clean the juicer after use to keep it operating efficiently. Use a small cleaning brush or even a toothbrush for this to get into all the crevices. It is simply a question of practice: you may find this task a little time-consuming initially, but eventually it will take you no more than five minutes. In any event, I would urge you always to clean the juicer before drinking your juice, otherwise the pulp will start to dry out and get stuck in the crevices. You will also feel less inclined to clean the juicer once the juice has been drunk.

WHICH INGREDIENTS DO YOU NEED TO PREPARE GREEN JUICES?

Once you are familiar with most of the positive effects of green juices and know which type of juicer best meets your personal requirements, all that is left for you to do is mix yourself a delicious juice and experience the beneficial effects for yourself.

But where to start? What are the main ingredients for green juices? The deeper you delve into the world of green juices, the more you will begin to create favorite mixes of your own and try out different ingredients. To get you started, here are a few basic rules for preparing a simple green juice:

RECIPE FORMULA FOR GREEN JUICES

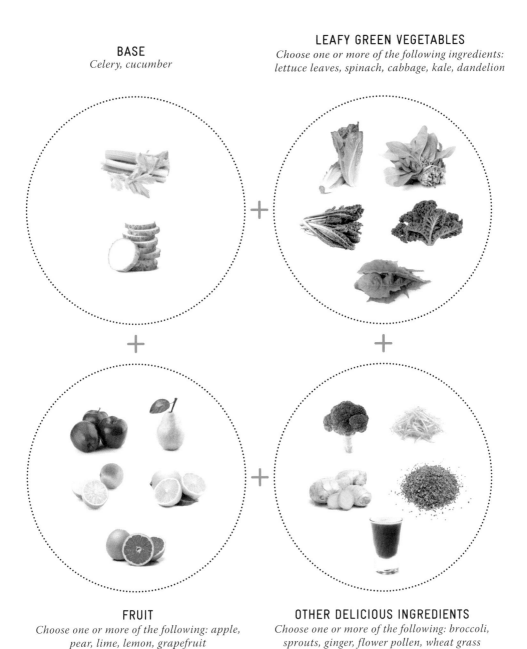

BASE
Celery, cucumber

LEAFY GREEN VEGETABLES
Choose one or more of the following ingredients:
lettuce leaves, spinach, cabbage, kale, dandelion

FRUIT
Choose one or more of the following: apple,
pear, lime, lemon, grapefruit

OTHER DELICIOUS INGREDIENTS
Choose one or more of the following: broccoli,
sprouts, ginger, flower pollen, wheat grass

1. "Green, how I love you, green!" (F. García Lorca in *Hypnotic Romance*): Choose one of the following: kale, spinach, lettuce, or Swiss chard.

2. Liquid: Take one or two of the following: celery, cucumber, or fennel.

3. Sweet note: Choose one or two of the following: lemon, lime, grapefruit, apple, or pear.

4. Topping: optional. Choose two or three of the following: ginger, broccoli, sprouts, flower pollen, wheat grass, or spirulina.

Preparation

1. Thoroughly clean the vegetables

One of my preferred methods of removing any dirt is to spray the ingredients using a bottle spray containing a mixture of one glass of water and two tablespoons of apple vinegar. Leave this mixture to work for five to ten minutes before rinsing in cold water. Root vegetables such as carrots or red beetroot are usually cleaned using a vegetable brush. This gets rid of any dirt or wax, but not chemical pesticides.

Vegetables for juicing should ideally be organically grown as the quality of organic vegetables and the amounts of micronutrients they contain differ considerably from vegetables grown in the conventional way. This also insures against us consuming any pesticides, herbicides, or other toxic substances which cannot be washed off and are harmful to the body.

If you do not use organic ingredients, I would recommend that you peel them. Although the peel may well contain many vitamins and minerals, it is also where the greatest concentration of residual chemical substances will be found (such as fertilizers, herbicides, pesticides …), and these will not be eliminated, no matter how thoroughly you spray the produce with vinegar. It follows, therefore, that green juices go very much hand in hand with organic products, although it is still better to drink green juice made from non-organic ingredients than none at all. The cleansing and purifying effect of green juices itself helps us to neutralize any harmful influences.

2. Cut up the ingredients

The size of the juicer's filler opening will dictate how small the chunks of fruit and vegetables need to be chopped.

3. Switch on the juicer and feed in the ingredients

I recommend alternating fibrous vegetables with less fibrous ones, for example, two stalks of celery followed by half a cucumber, so that the juicer does not become clogged up and the ingredients get pushed to the bottom. Pass the pulp through the juicer one more time to extract the last drops of juice.

Depending on the juicer model, this can take between five seconds and five minutes.

4. Sieve the juice

This step is optional. Even with a juice extractor, residual bits of pulp will often remain in the juice. If you want your juice to be 100 percent liquid, you will need to strain the juice through a very fine sieve or piece of cheesecloth.

Tip for making a thinner juice: add a little water or coconut water.

Sugar content in green juice

Are you in the mood for a carrot, apple, orange, or pineapple drink? Who could refuse something so sweet and delicious? You should bear in mind, however, that fruit—and to a lesser extent root vegetables such as beetroot and carrots—contains a good deal of sugar. When making juice, we discard the fibers, but these are actually what help slow down sugar absorption into the body. Without fibers, the sugar is quickly absorbed and will cause a rapid increase in blood-sugar levels and, consequently, a hefty insulin reaction (insulin is the hormone which regulates blood sugar). If the body's insulin levels regularly rise sharply, this can cause a metabolic imbalance, leading to diabetes and weight increase. The best fruits to add to vegetable juices are therefore those with a low sugar content, such as green apples, green pears, lemons, limes, or grapefruit. As Dr. Norman Walker, the pioneer of vegetable juices and healthy diet, remarked so appositely: "Drink your vegetables and eat your fruit."

After all, we drink green juices in order to bring our health into balance. For this reason, I always advise adding leafy greens to the juices and, if using a mixture of several types of fruit or vegetables, drinking the juice either before engaging in sport or at breakfast time when there is still the whole morning left during which to burn up the sugar.

People who suffer from diabetes or candidiasis can still enjoy these wonderful green juices as long as they do not contain any root vegetables or any fruits other than lemons, limes, or grapefruit.

Ringing the changes with leafy greens

You may now be wondering: what is wrong with mixing two handfuls of spinach with my green juice every morning? If this is what you have been doing until now, then don't worry. However, it is a good idea and advisable to ring the changes with regard to which types of leafy vegetables you use. My two main reasons for this are as follows:

1. Avoiding the toxic effects of anti-nutrients

All green leaves contain a substance which protects them from predators. Spinach, for example, contains oxalic acid, which can cause problems for people who are prone to kidney stones. The vegetable family of crucifers (kale and other types of cabbage, broccoli, cauliflower ...) contain goitrogens, substances which can affect the function of the thyroid gland in some people.

If you are in good health and frequently consume these types of vegetable, you need not worry. It is most unlikely that these substances would reach harmful levels if your diet is healthy and balanced. However, if you are healthy but follow a raw-food diet and consume two or three portions of leafy greens on a daily basis, it is important to vary the types of vegetable regularly.

2. Getting a good range of nutrients

Put simply, different types of vegetables provide us with different nutrients in varying concentrations. Kale, for example, contains more iron and calcium than spinach; rucola provides us with more vitamin A and C than lettuce.

It is advisable therefore to choose different varieties of green-leaf vegetables and ring the changes (as vegetables belonging to the same plant family will contain the same anti-nutrients and have very similar nutritional values). Below is a short summary:

– Brassicaceae/crucifers: kale, other types of cabbage, cauliflower, pak choi, rucola, broccoli, radish, and mustard leaves.
– Asteraceae: all types of lettuce and dandelion.
– Amaranthaceae: spinach, Swiss chard, red beetroot leaves.
– Apiaceae: celery, cilantro, parsley, carrot leaves.

How to economize when buying ingredients

Consuming green juices on a daily basis will inevitably have implications for your finances. Nevertheless, it is without doubt the best investment you could possibly make for the sake of your health. In my household we live by the principle that "health is priceless!" And this is perfectly true, since it is virtually impossible to imagine what we would do if we did not have our health. At the same time, we must also be practical and realistic and, like you, I prefer not to spend more than I have to on food purchases if I can reduce costs using a few little tricks:

Shopping at local markets

Seasonal vegetables are often up to 50 percent cheaper here than at the supermarket. If you shop regularly at a particular stall, you may even build up such a good relationship with the local producer that you are offered a discount or an extra vegetable or two for good measure.

Buying large quantities on special offer

This may not be possible with every kind of vegetable, but it is certainly a good idea for the ones you use most frequently, for example, lettuce, apples, celery, etc. ... Buying them in larger quantities will save you money and also act as an incentive to make yourself a green juice every day. As a result, the ingredients are unlikely to go off.

Do not buy packs of pre-washed or pre-sliced vegetables

These will be much more expensive than loose vegetables and are never as fresh. What is more, the packaging and bags used for prepared produce also contain preservative gases to keep the product fresh for longer.

Buying seasonal produce

As a rule, these products are cheaper because they are produced in increased quantities at particular times of the year. Apples are cheaper during winter, whereas cucumbers cost less than half as much in summer as they do at other times of the year. Vary your choice of vegetables depending on the season: use more kale in the winter months, for example, and lettuce during the summer.

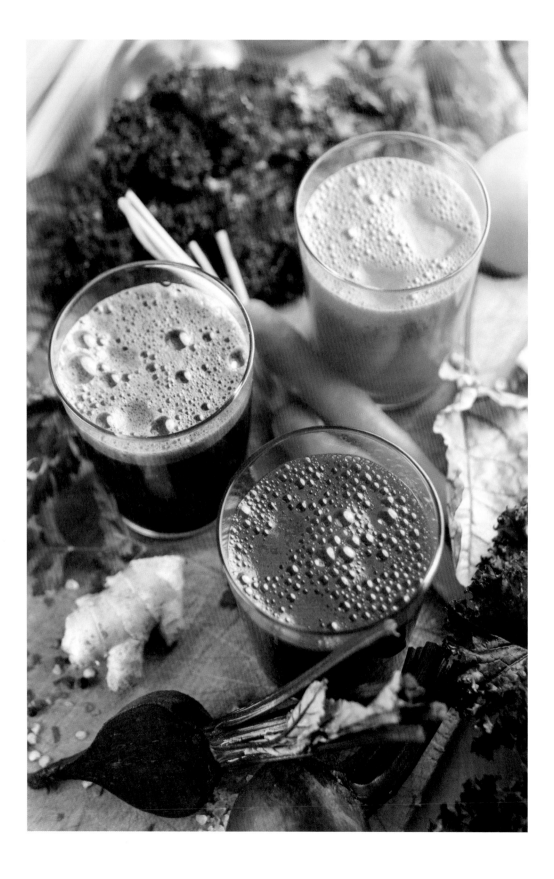

THE MOST COMMON INGREDIENTS IN GREEN JUICES

Green juices are always made from the same basic ingredients, as it is these which provide the health benefits we hope to derive from drinking vegetable juice. All the ingredients not only have strong alkalizing and hydrating properties, but also contain large amounts of vitamins and minerals. Each ingredient will be described in detail over the following pages.

KALE

PROPERTIES

– The mineral levels in cabbage are perfectly balanced. As a result, the calcium it contains is more readily absorbed by the body than the calcium contained in milk. Kale is therefore good for promoting healthy bones and considered particularly useful in preventing osteoporosis.

– Because of its acid-neutralizing and anti-inflammatory properties, kale is one of the best natural acid regulators. In its raw juice form, it is ideal for treating stomach and duodenal ulcers as well as inflammatory bowel disorders.

– It is also believed to possess anti-carcinogenic properties.

– It also helps to disperse the build-up of fluids in the body and is therefore very effective in the treatment of diabetes, obesity, gout, and heart disease which may also be accompanied by increased fluid retention.

– It belongs to the family of crucifers and consequently affects the production of hormones by the thyroid gland, which is why excessive consumption of this vegetable is not recommended for people with an over- or under-active thyroid.

....

Kale—originally a cultivar of the wild cabbage found in Southern and Western Europe – has been grown in Europe for centuries. It has meanwhile also become very popular in the USA. As well as all the usual substances found in cabbage varieties it also contains a large amount of iron.

....

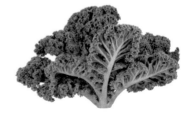

VITAMIN AND MINERAL CONTENT

– Kale is rich in vitamin A and C. It also contains folic acid (vitamin B9) and vitamin B3. Potassium and calcium are the main minerals found in kale, followed by phosphorus and magnesium.

DANDELION

PROPERTIES

- The tender young leaves of the dandelion plant are rich in nutrients. They are also great for detoxing, cleansing, and strengthening the blood and are highly recommended in the treatment of anemia. Dandelion increases the production of red blood corpuscles, reduces uric acid, and regulates blood pressure.

- It has diuretic properties which stimulate and cleanse the kidneys, which is why it is highly recommended in the treatment of urinary-tract infections and kidney stones. Whereas other diuretics cause loss of calcium, dandelion does not reduce the body's calcium content.

- Dandelion juice has a bitter taste, stimulates bile flow, and relieves blockages in the liver. It has mildly digestive properties and can help alleviate constipation. It can also stimulate appetite and relieve upset stomachs.

- It is very effective in the treatment of skin disorders such as psoriasis, skin rashes, or eczema.

- Dandelion is also recommended in the treatment of arthritis, rheumatism, and other chronic joint diseases. It regulates menstruation problems and stimulates the production of breast milk.

Everyone will have blown the seeds off a dandelion globe as a child. The plant gets its name from its serrated leaves, which resemble the pointed irregular teeth of a lion.

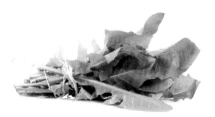

VITAMIN AND MINERAL CONTENT

- Dandelions contain high concentrations of vitamin A, B-group vitamins (especially folic acid), and vitamins C and D. They are also full of iron and have high levels of calcium, potassium, zinc, and copper.

SPINACH

PROPERTIES
- Thanks to its high iron content, regular consumption of spinach increases the hemoglobin content in the blood.
- Spinach protects the stomach lining, thereby helping to prevent stomach ulcers.
- It also helps prevent vitamin A deficiency, itching and dry eyes, and eye ulcers.
- It contains antioxidants which strengthen muscles, especially the heart muscles; it consequently protects against heart and circulatory problems, high blood pressure, and arteriosclerosis.

VITAMIN AND MINERAL CONTENT
- In addition to its remarkably high protein content, spinach is also an excellent natural source of vitamins and minerals. In terms of vitamin content, it is rich in vitamins A, C, E, and K as well as B-group vitamins (B6, B2, B1) and folic acid (vitamin B9).
- The main minerals found in spinach include calcium, iron, potassium, magnesium, manganese, and phosphorus.

Despite the controversy surrounding the naturally high levels of histamine in spinach, it still remains one of the top vegetables in any vegan diet. Its protein and iron concentrations are among the highest found in any leaf vegetable.

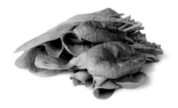

LETTUCE

PROPERTIES

- Lettuce is known to have a tranquilizing effect on the human body. It helps to calm the nerves and control palpitations, which is why it is especially recommended for sleep disorders.

- If consumed before meals—whether in a salad or in juice form—it will strengthen the stomach and improve digestion.

- Lettuce is recommended in the case of renal insufficiency as its diuretic properties help stimulate kidney function. Its diuretic effect in conjunction with its high fiber content will help to reduce blood-sugar levels. Lettuce is therefore highly recommended for people suffering from diabetes.

- Lettuce improves circulation, prevents arteriosclerosis, and reduces cholesterol levels in the blood.

- During pregnancy, lettuce is an excellent source of folic acid—folic acid is very important for fetal development.

When choosing different types of lettuce, we should remember that some varieties have had their natural bitterness cultivated out; these generally contain a large amount of water but little in the way of nutritional value. As a general rule, the more bitter varieties and those with strongly colored leaves tend to contain the most chlorophyll, nutrients, and antioxidants.

VITAMIN AND MINERAL CONTENT

- Lettuce contains large quantities of antioxidants: beta-carotene and vitamins C and E. It also has an exceptionally high folic acid content (vitamin B9).

- Lettuce is particularly rich in potassium; it also supplies calcium, phosphorus, selenium, and bromine. The latter is known to be beneficial in treating nervous conditions.

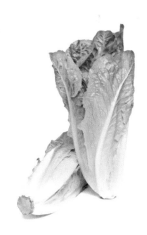

29

MINT

PROPERTIES

- Mint leaves are rich in chlorophyll, which, as already mentioned, is a very effective blood-cleansing and -regenerating substance. For this reason, mint is regarded as a medicinal plant and a star ingredient in green juices.
- This plant is extremely useful in aiding digestion. It stimulates the liver and bile flow, thereby encouraging the digestion of fats. Mint is also good for preventing bad breath.
- Its anti-flatulent properties also help the dispersal of accumulated intestinal gases.
- Mint's high concentrations of menthol act as a decongestant on the respiratory passages and also have anti-viral properties. Mint also works as an expectorant on the bronchial passages, helping to loosen coughs.
- Thanks to its anti-coagulant properties, mint improves blood circulation by thinning the blood.

VITAMIN AND MINERAL CONTENT

- Mint contains vitamin C, vitamin A, and B-group vitamins, especially vitamin B9 or folic acid.
- It provides us with minerals in the form of potassium, calcium, magnesium, phosphorus, zinc, and iron.

Mint has long been reputed to be an aphrodisiac. It was also used by the ancient Greeks to freshen the air in their homes and to perfume bath water.

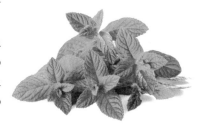

PARSLEY

PROPERTIES

– Parsley has a very high concentration of chlorophyll and has a powerful cleansing effect, although one of its essential oils can be toxic if consumed in excessive amounts. Its high vitamin C content boosts the immune system and, in conjunction with the high flavonoid content, increases the blood's anti-oxidative powers.

– The addition of parsley to green juice or to food dishes has proved to be extremely beneficial in aiding digestion as it supports the stomach and acts as an anti-flatulent by reducing the amount of gases. It also soothes stomachache and intestinal cramps.

– Eating parsley in combination with other iron-rich vegetables is highly recommended for anyone suffering from anemia as its folic acid and vitamin C content encourages the body's absorption of iron.

– Parsley is a powerful diuretic plant which can prevent the formation of kidney stones and alleviates menstrual pain. It is also a useful plant during the menopause as it stimulates estrogen production.

VITAMIN AND MINERAL CONTENT

– Parsley has particularly high concentrations of vitamin C, vitamin A, folic acid (vitamin B9), and vitamin K, which plays a major role in blood-clotting. The main minerals in parsley are potassium, calcium, magnesium, and iron.

....
How did the healthy practice of using parsley as a garnish for certain dishes first arise? If you read up on its many beneficial properties, you will soon understand why and keep a parsley plant on your own window sill.
....

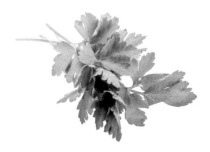

CELERY

PROPERTIES

- Celery is an effective diuretic and excellent blood purifier. It contains large quantities of minerals, which also have a strong re-mineralizing effect. Thanks to its high vitamin C content, this nutrient is also a very good antioxidant.

- Regular consumption of celery will help to reduce the blood's cholesterol levels, and its anti-inflammatory properties make it a good ally in conjunction with anti-cancer diets. In Ayurvedic medicine, it is frequently used to combat rheumatic diseases. It can also be very good for the digestive system. Its high fiber content helps to alleviate chronic constipation.

VITAMIN AND MINERAL CONTENT

- Celery consists of 95 percent water, which is why it can be very useful if you are trying to lose weight. It is also rich in vitamins and minerals, especially vitamin C and B-group vitamins. Celery is a very important source of potassium; it also supplies us with phosphorus, calcium, magnesium, and iron.

Celery has a bitter-sweet flavor which makes it a refreshing ingredient. Its high water content and strong alkalizing properties make it a star ingredient.

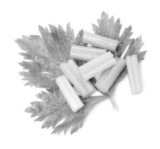

CUCUMBER

PROPERTIES

- Regardless of whether they are eaten—especially the peel—or used externally, cucumbers regulate the acid content of the skin and restore its balance.
- The juices released during chewing are good for healing and soothing inflamed gums. Phytochemical substances found in cucumbers are also useful for keeping breath fresh.
- Thanks to their high water content and large amounts of phytonutrients, cucumbers have powerful purifying properties and help to fight diabetes, lower cholesterol levels, and regulate blood pressure.
- The fact that cucumbers have a high water content and are low in calories makes them an ideal food for anyone wishing to lose weight. The high fiber content is also beneficial to the digestive processes. Eating cucumber on a daily basis will help to prevent chronic constipation.

VITAMIN AND MINERAL CONTENT

- Cucumber contains vitamins A, B, and C, all of which support the immune system and supply energy. To increase the effectiveness of cucumber in this respect, its juice can be mixed with that of spinach and carrots. Do not peel the cucumber, as its skin contains 12 percent of our daily vitamin C requirement.
- Cucumber also contains vitamin K, which is known for its anti-inflammatory and anti-hemorrhagic properties.
- The main minerals contained in cucumbers are potassium, magnesium, and silicon.

....
Cucumber and celery are two of the basic ingredients in green juice. Both provide exactly the right kind of fluid to create the perfect consistency of a good juice. Cucumbers are also greatly valued as an ingredient in natural cosmetics: even Cleopatra used them as part of her beauty regime.
....

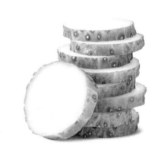

LEMONS

PROPERTIES

- Lemons stimulate bile flow in people suffering from liver or gall-bladder problems, thereby encouraging fat metabolism.

- By removing toxins from the blood plasma, lemons can do much to support the heart and circulatory system, especially in people suffering from arteriosclerosis or high blood pressure. They are equally effective in the case of rheumatic diseases such as gout, as they can get rid of crystallized toxins from the joints.

- Their high vitamin C concentrations help increase iron absorption when combined with other ingredients. They also increase the fruit's refreshing, antiseptic, anti-bacterial, and anti-viral properties, which can alleviate certain diseases of the respiratory tract, including inflammation of the vocal chords or tonsils.

- Despite their extremely sour taste, lemons have a strong alkalizing effect on the body.

VITAMIN AND MINERAL CONTENT

- In addition to vitamin C, lemons also contain vitamin B-group vitamins and vitamin E, as well as a large number of minerals: potassium, magnesium, calcium, phosphorus, copper, zinc, iron, and manganese. This cocktail of vitamins and minerals also helps boost the immune system.

Although lemons are known for their high vitamin C content, what really distinguishes this fruit is its ability to neutralize and eliminate toxins in our body. Lemons have strong alkalizing properties, are good at removing toxins, and are wonderfully purifying. Regularly drinking a glass of lukewarm water mixed with the juice of a lemon will help to get rid of toxins and fortify the liver.

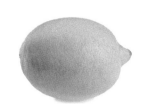

APPLE

PROPERTIES

- The potassium contained in apples makes the fruit mildly diuretic and is ideal for people suffering from water retention and/or kidney-function problems.

- Rich in antioxidants and flavonoids, apples protect the cells from attack by free radicals. This, combined with their ability to neutralize toxins, makes apples a significant cancer-inhibiting food. Their cleansing properties are equally valuable in treating gout (an excess of uric acid in the blood), rheumatic diseases, and obesity.

- Eating a few bites of a good apple each day will help to prevent tooth decay as apples reduce the number of bacteria in the mouth.

- Apple peel contains non-soluble fibers which help prevent constipation. Grated apple, on the other hand, which has been exposed to the air, can be useful in treating diarrhea.

VITAMIN AND MINERAL CONTENT

- Apples have a high vitamin C content, which is why they are also a rich source of antioxidants as well as B-group vitamins. The main minerals in apples are calcium, phosphorus, and potassium. They are also rich in soluble and insoluble fibers.

The apple, which was considered a forbidden fruit until Eve did us the favor of biting into one, is one of the best fruits for purifying purposes. As the saying goes: "an apple a day keeps the doctor away."

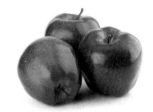

PEARS

PROPERTIES

- Because of their high water and fiber content and their low calorie count, pears are an ideal fruit to help you lose weight. They help to keep the stomach feeling full, purify the body, and at the same time regulate bowel function.

- They have a low glycemic index, a fact which, combined with their high potassium and low sodium content and pectin levels (water-soluble fiber), makes them very useful to anyone suffering from diabetes, raised cholesterol levels, high blood pressure or heart and circulatory problems in general.

- Because of their high folic acid content, which is very important in the development of babies, pears are a highly recommended food during pregnancy and breast-feeding.

- Furthermore, thanks to high tannin levels, pears also have anti-bacterial and anti-inflammatory properties which are very useful in combatting or relieving herpes blisters.

VITAMIN AND MINERAL CONTENT

- Pears contain many different vitamins (A, B1, B2, C, and E) and are also a source of folic acid (vitamin B9).

- It is likewise a good source of minerals such as potassium, phosphorus, calcium, magnesium, selenium, and iron; the last of these boosts red blood corpuscles.

Because of their mild flavor and the fact that they rarely trigger allergic reactions, pears are ideal as a first food for babies who are being weaned off breast milk and consequently may well be a baby's first introduction to green juice.

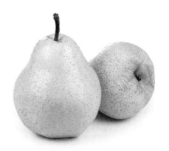

GRAPEFRUIT

PROPERTIES

- Grapefruit is a natural, nutritious, low-calorie food.

- Its abundant supply of antioxidants such as vitamin C makes it a very effective factor in the prevention of cancer as it gets rid of free radicals which attack cell DNA and are responsible for oxidative stress.

- It can also help to prevent the formation of or even dissolve kidney stones as well as stimulate and boost the immune system. Eating grapefruit is consequently recommended as a natural defense measure against the common cold and a good way to maintain a healthy regime during the colds and flu season.

- A study published in the *Journal of Agricultural and Food Chemistry*, carried out on 57 patients who had undergone bypass surgery, showed that, in just one month, regular consumption of grapefruit resulted in a significant reduction in cholesterol levels and triglycerides.

VITAMIN AND MINERAL CONTENT

- The predominant nutrients in grapefruit include high levels of vitamin C, folic acid (vitamin B9), anti-oxidative carotenoids (vitamin A), potassium, and magnesium.

- It also contains much smaller quantities of vitamin B2, vitamin B1, iron, calcium, and phosphorus.

Did you know that grapefruit can be very helpful if you are trying to lose weight? Its diuretic properties help get rid of excess fluids. It also contains many enzymes which help to stabilize blood-sugar and insulin levels. This makes us feel much more energetic and less hungry between meals.

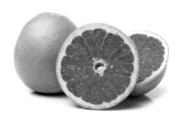

WATERMELON

PROPERTIES

- Watermelons are low in fat and calories, but contain abundant phytonutrients and antioxidants, which are essential for optimal health.

- The high content of lycopene and other antioxidants in a watermelon make it a super-fruit in terms of fighting inflammatory conditions and free radicals. A glass of watermelon juice each day can reduce the risk of diseases such as rheumatoid arthritis, asthma, and bowel cancer.

- Because of their high water content, watermelons are highly recommended for purifying the kidneys and bladder. Their high concentration of potassium also reduces uric acid in the blood and helps to get rid of toxins from the kidneys.

- They help to break down deposits within the arteries and also keep eyes healthy.

  They eliminate the factors which can cause muscle fatigue and help prepare the muscles to start producing more energy again. Drinking watermelon juice after intense physical activity is a quick and natural way of restoring muscle function.

VITAMIN AND MINERAL CONTENT

- Watermelon consists of 90 percent water. Even so, it is an abundant source of vitamins A and C. It has a high potassium content and also contains magnesium, calcium, and phosphorus.

Hieroglyphics and sculptures from ancient Egypt show that watermelons were already being cultivated in the Nile Valley around 3,500 years ago. Square and heart-shaped water melons are now also available on the Japanese market.

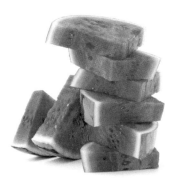

BROCCOLI

PROPERTIES

– Broccoli is one of the most important vegetables in an anti-cancer diet. It is a rich source of antioxidants which help to eliminate toxins, free radicals, and uric acid, thereby cleansing the blood. Its vitamin C content is also important for boosting the immune system.

– Broccoli belongs to the family of crucifers and therefore contains substances which inhibit thyroid function. Anyone suffering from a thyroid imbalance is advised to limit their broccoli consumption.

– It is a source of easily absorbable calcium and magnesium, thereby helping to support bone health.

– Because of its folic acid content, which is important for fetal development, broccoli is highly recommended during pregnancy.

– Its high iron content also makes it especially useful for anemia sufferers.

– In addition, it helps to promote healthy skin and hair.

VITAMIN AND MINERAL CONTENT

– Broccoli is an excellent source of vitamin C, as well as B-group vitamins and vitamins A and E. The main minerals in broccoli are potassium and calcium. It also supplies decent amounts of magnesium, phosphorus, and iron.

An old home remedy for preventing the odor of broccoli permeating the entire house during cooking was to add a slice of bread to the saucepan.

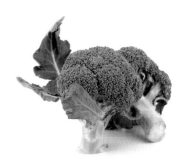

ONIONS

PROPERTIES

- The onion, along with garlic, is one of our best natural antibiotics; the bactericidal components found in onions are the best natural defense against infections. Onions are also good for treating coughs.

- Onions also contain anti-thrombotic properties which are useful for reducing high blood pressure and thinning the blood. They can also help to prevent allergic reactions caused by pollen.

- Onions aid the digestive processes by stimulating the liver, gall bladder, and pancreas. They also help to alleviate symptoms of inflammatory bowel disease such as Crohn's or celiac disease.

- Recent studies have shown that tumor-inhibiting effects in anti-cancer treatment may be ascribed to the regular consumption of onions.

- Onions are also important diuretics and therefore highly recommended for helping to getting rid of excess fluids caused by overweight, rheumatism, gout, or kidney failure. They also help to prevent osteoporosis.

Onions contain sulfur which is released when the onions are cut open, and it is this which makes us cry. Simply think of them as tears of joy— they do, after all, bring countless benefits for your health.

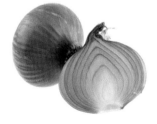

VITAMIN AND MINERAL CONTENT

- Onions contain vitamin C and B-group vitamins. They are also an excellent source of potassium, sulfur (the substance responsible for its anti-bacterial properties), phosphorus, calcium, and magnesium.

ASPARAGUS

PROPERTIES

- As an excellent source not only of antioxidants in general but also of folic acid, vitamin A, and zinc, asparagus—along with red beetroot—is one of the best anti-aging foods available.

- It contains cellulose, which is indigestible and therefore stimulates the large intestine, relieving constipation.

- Asparagus is one of the most powerful diuretics in the vegetable world and is consequently excellent for lowering blood pressure. It is common knowledge that eating asparagus causes urine to smell stronger, but this is a perfectly harmless side-effect.

- Asparagus is ideal for alleviating tiredness and stress situations.

- The beta-carotene and vitamin C contained in asparagus are antioxidants which help to fight cancer, heart disease, and eye problems.

VITAMIN AND MINERAL CONTENT

- Asparagus contains large amounts of vitamins A, C , and E; it also has significant levels of B-group vitamins, especially vitamins B9 (folic acid) and B2 (riboflavin).

- The main minerals in asparagus are potassium, calcium, phosphorus, magnesium, iron, and zinc.

Hippocrates himself recommended tea made from dried asparagus as a diuretic drink. It has been used as a medicinal plant since the Middle Ages, and its remedial properties have been described in medicinal herb books since the 15th century.

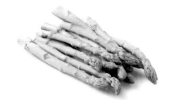

FENNEL

PROPERTIES

- Fennel is a good source of phytoestrogens, which work in women like natural estrogen, and has been used for centuries to help regulate menstruation. It is also rich in antioxidants, which combat the cell-destroying effects of free radicals. It is known to have a beneficial effect on the heart and circulatory system by lowering blood pressure and reducing cholesterol, among other things.

- Fennel also has antibacterial properties which are very efficient in countering bad breath, gum disease, bowel bacteria and parasites, and infections. It simultaneously improves digestion and alleviates stomach problems. It also acts as an expectorant and can help to improve vision. Fennel stimulates milk flow in nursing mothers.

VITAMIN AND MINERAL CONTENT

- Fennel is especially rich in vitamin C and also contains lesser amounts of B-group vitamins, the main one of which is folic acid.

- The main minerals in fennel are potassium, calcium, phosphorus, and magnesium.

This medicinal plant has a similar flavor to that of aniseed. All parts of the plant are edible: the root, stem, leaves, flowers, fruits, and seeds. Fennel has figured in superstition since Roman times. The ancient Romans believed that a few sprigs of fennel in the kitchen would give protection from all kinds of diseases.

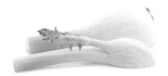

RED BELL PEPPER

PROPERTIES

- Red bell peppers help to preserve healthy vision, especially night vision; they are also good for the skin, hair, and fingernails.

- This vegetable has one of the highest levels of lycopene, a substance which has been found in tests to be successful in preventing cancer, especially of the prostate or lungs.

- As a good source of carotenoids, this vegetable can help to fight inflammatory ailments and pain since it acts as an analgesic.

VITAMIN AND MINERAL CONTENT

- In addition to its high lycopene content, red bell pepper is an important source of vitamins C and A. It also supplies us with B vitamins, especially vitamin B6.

- The main mineral contained in red peppers is potassium. However, they also contain calcium, phosphorus, and magnesium. The natural balance between these three minerals in red bell peppers helps maintain healthy bones and tissue.

Did you know that green peppers are unripe red peppers? This is why they have a slightly bitter flavor and, compared to red peppers, contain only half as much vitamin C and a tenth of the amount of vitamin A.

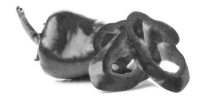

RADISH VARIETIES

PROPERTIES

- Radishes are regarded quite simply as a super-vegetable, effective in fighting all kinds of diseases: they have anti-carcinogenic, anti-inflammatory, and anti-microbial properties.

- They regulate bowel function, alleviate digestive problems, and also help to fight infection and colds. They can relieve the symptoms of rheumatism and gout and can help in the treatment of ulcers.

- They can stimulate bile production, thereby helping to process fat into usable energy and eliminate waste products and toxins from the body.

- Rich in iodine, radishes helps maintain thyroid function, which regulates metabolism and is important for growth.

VITAMIN AND MINERAL CONTENT

- Radishes consist of nearly 95 percent water, containing hardly any proteins, fats, or carbohydrates. The radish is also one of the best sources of vitamin C of any vegetable and is also known for its significant folic acid (vitamin B9) content.

- The main minerals contained in radishes are potassium and iodine. Potassium plays a key role in transmitting nerve impulses as well as in maintaining normal muscle activity.

Despite the little saying we have in Spanish—when something is of no interest—that we do "not care a radish about something," radishes do, in fact, interest us greatly. A vegetable which has such a high, positive impact on our health cannot be ignored.

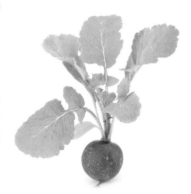

RED BEETROOT

PROPERTIES

- The high sugar and iron content in red beetroot makes it an excellent source of energy and extremely useful in aiding the treatment of anemia and blood disorders, and during convalescence.

- Rich in flavonoids, it has been seen to act as an effective anti-carcinogenic.

- Beetroot is a strongly alkaline vegetable. It supports the liver in its role as a detoxifier by neutralizing acid in the body.

- It is highly recommended during pregnancy on account of its high folic acid content, which, as has been mentioned several times, is crucial for fetal development.

- As an excellent source of soluble and insoluble fiber, it is also well known for its powerful cleansing properties.

- It also has diuretic properties which help to rid the body of excess fluids.

All parts of the beetroot plant can be utilized; its leaves are a good source of vitamin A and excellent for stimulating the digestive processes. When nutrients are in juice form, compounds can form which make these nutrients easier to absorb. Such is the case with beetroot and iron, since the iron found in beetroot juice is much more easily absorbed than other forms of iron.

VITAMIN AND MINERAL CONTENT

- Because of its starch content, beetroot's carbohydrates are reabsorbed slowly. The root contains a large amount of vitamin C and lots of B vitamins, especially folic acid (vitamin B9).

- With regard to minerals, beetroot is rich in iodine and potassium. It also contains smaller amounts of magnesium, phosphorus, and calcium.

- Beetroot leaves are rich in beta-carotene and minerals such as iron and calcium.

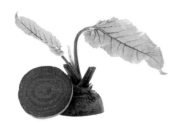

TOMATOES

PROPERTIES

- Tomatoes are a rich source of antioxidants, containing large amounts of lycopene, an extremely effective antioxidant against cancer caused by free radicals (especially prostate cancer).

- They reduce cholesterol levels and protect the heart. Eating tomatoes on a daily basis will reduce the risk of high blood pressure.

- Tomatoes encourage a healthy digestive system and prevent constipation; they have a laxative effect, particularly if eaten with the skin intact although tomato pips and skin can also aggravate sensitive stomachs.

- They are also an efficient aid in helping the body to get rid of toxins and heavy metals. Regular consumption reduces the occurrence of urinary-tract infections and bladder cancer.

- Vitamin A contained in tomatoes helps to improve vision and prevents night blindness. Medical studies have also shown that including tomatoes in one's daily diet reduces oxidative stress in Type-2 diabetes cases.

Tomato juice stimulates digestion, balances out nutrient levels, is good for blood function, and has interesting regeneration properties. It is not recommended for people suffering from stomach ache, but it is good for boosting weak immune systems.

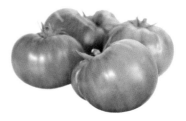

VITAMIN AND MINERAL CONTENT

- Tomatoes contain numerous vitamins: vitamin A, vitamin C and B vitamins, plus a certain amount of vitamins E, P, and D.

- They are rich in potassium, phosphorus, calcium and magnesium. They also contain smaller amounts of manganese, zinc, and copper.

CARROTS

PROPERTIES

– Regular consumption of carrots, whether in a salad, juice, or purée, increases the body's red blood corpuscle count and hemoglobin. The latter is regarded as an important regulator in maintaining a healthy acid–alkaline balance in the body.

– Eating carrots on a regular basis helps to alleviate stomach and duodenal ulcers as they build up the stomach's muscle tissue.

– Their high carotene content not only helps us to tan safely and more quickly, but also protects us from cancer, especially pancreatic cancer. Carotenoids also protect the arteries and immune system and help fight infections.

– For nursing mothers, carrots improve the biological quality of breast milk.

– They improve the health and appearance of hair and nails and are very effective in maintaining good vision.

It is now fashionable to cultivate a colorful range of carrots, and you can now find white, yellow, dark-red, and purple carrots available in shops, ideal for making salads or colorful juice mixtures. The leaves can likewise go straight into the juicer. Each green leaf is a valuable addition to a purifying green juice because of its high chlorophyll content.

VITAMIN AND MINERAL CONTENT

– Like beetroot, carrots contain a large amount of starch, which changes carbohydrates into slowly reabsorbable sugar. In addition to their high carotene content, carrots also provide us with a remarkable number of minerals, such as calcium, iron, potassium and phosphorus, as well as vitamins B, C, and D.

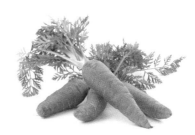

GARLIC

PROPERTIES

- Garlic is often used for its cough-suppressant and natural antibiotic properties.

- It contains alliin, a substance which lowers blood pressure and stimulates the circulatory system.

- It has strong diuretic properties which help alleviate water retention. It is therefore highly recommended in the treatment of obesity, rheumatism, arthritis, or gout.

- Because of its high levels of flavonoids, antioxidants, and sulfur compounds, it is useful as an anti-carcinogenic.

Garlic has been famed for its healing properties since the days of ancient Egypt, Greece, and Rome. To be effective garlic should be eaten raw. Adding it to our juice mixtures will preserve its beneficial properties.

VITAMIN AND MINERAL CONTENT

- Garlic is rich in vitamin C and vitamin B6. It also contains smaller amounts of folic acid (vitamin B9) and vitamin B3.

- It also contains relatively high amounts of the following minerals: potassium, calcium and phosphorus, as well as smaller amounts of magnesium, iron, and copper.

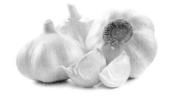

GINGER

PROPERTIES

– Ginger helps to increase the amount of intestinal flora, or "good bacteria." It acts as a natural antibiotic which is able to fight infectious bacteria.

– It stimulates the pancreas and the production of digestive enzymes which help the digestive processes.

– Ginger boosts body heat. It also aids blood circulation, can dissolve clots in the arteries, and can lower cholesterol levels. It is effective against nausea, dizziness, and faintness, and is very useful for fighting viral infections in the upper respiratory tract, such as sinusitis, colds, and flu.

– Ginger root is a spice which is highly recommended for the treatment of depression and for lifting spirits as it stimulates the production of endorphins, commonly known as "happy hormones."

VITAMIN AND MINERAL CONTENT

– Ginger is a good source of vitamin A, vitamin C, and vitamins B1, B2, and B6. Its mineral content includes potassium, calcium, magnesium, phosphorus, and iron.

The root is the only part of the plant that is eaten. Originating in the Far East, ginger was as valuable a commodity as silk and was transported to the West along hundreds of kilometers of trade routes. It has an exotic history extending over several centuries.

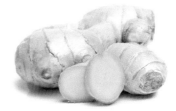

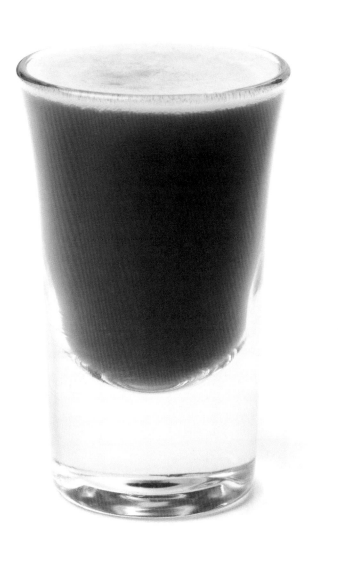

GREEN JUICE RECIPES

The following pages contain a collection of 30 recipes for green and not-so-green juices, all of which have alkalizing, purifying, and regenerating properties. The names I have given the different juice recipes also give an indication of the kind of positive effect you can expect from each juice.

I hope that you will enjoy every single one of the following recipes and feel inspired to try out recipes of your own.

Enjoy!

*Always wash the vegetables thoroughly—see page 20!

GLORIOUS MORNING

*A feel-good and energy-boosting drink
to start the day*

INGREDIENTS

1 apple
½ cucumber
2 celery stalks
*5 sprigs of parsley or
cilantro*
1 handful of spinach
*1 piece of ginger
(thumbnail-sized)*

PREPARATION

Wash and drain the vegetables, then pat dry with a cloth or paper towel. If you are using organic vegetables, there is no need to peel. Otherwise, peel the apple and cucumber. Cut everything into pieces small enough to fit through the filler opening in the juicer.

Add the ingredients to the juicer one by one until the juice is ready.

Drink and enjoy immediately!

EFFECT

This juice is the perfect green drink to replace coffee and get the day off to a good start. Drinking a liter or more of this each day will discourage unhealthy snacking between meals.

This energy-boosting green juice also has cleansing and diuretic properties.

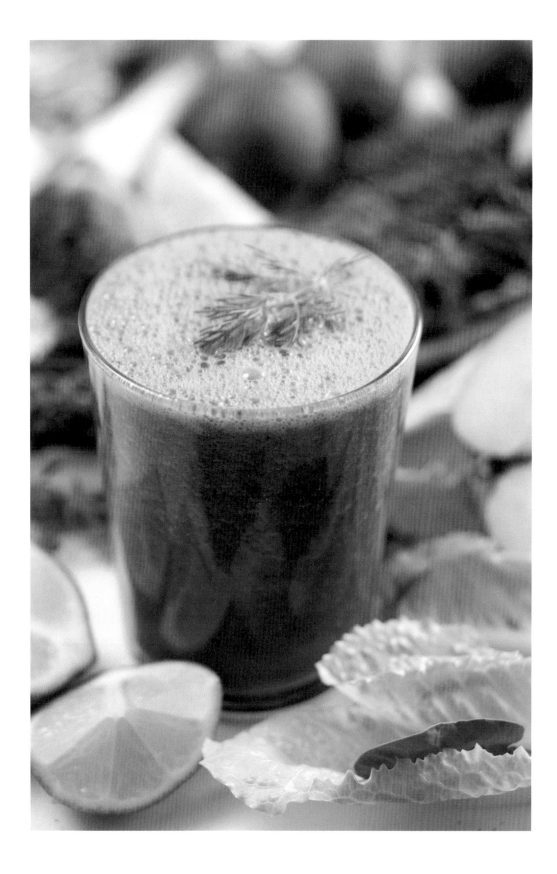

GOOD MORNING

*A sweet juice to start the day with a powerful energy boost
and leave you feeling pleasantly full*

INGREDIENTS

1 apple
2 carrots
½ cucumber
2 celery stalks
½ pineapple

PREPARATION

Wash all the ingredients except for the pineapple, then pat dry using a cloth or paper towel. If you are using organic produce, there is no need to peel. Otherwise peel the apple, carrots, and cucumber. Peel and chop the pineapple. Chop everything into pieces small enough to fit through the filler opening of the juicer. Feed the ingredients into the juicer one by one until the juice is ready.

Drink and enjoy immediately!

EFFECT

This recipe is perfect for beginners: the juice mixture is very mild and palatable because of its predominantly sweet flavor. It is ideal for getting used to green juices without compromising on flavor. The carrots add an extra portion of anti-oxidative beta-carotenes, whilst pineapple intensifies the drink's diuretic and filling properties. Anyone suffering from diabetes or candidiasis is advised to select a green juice recipe containing less fruit.

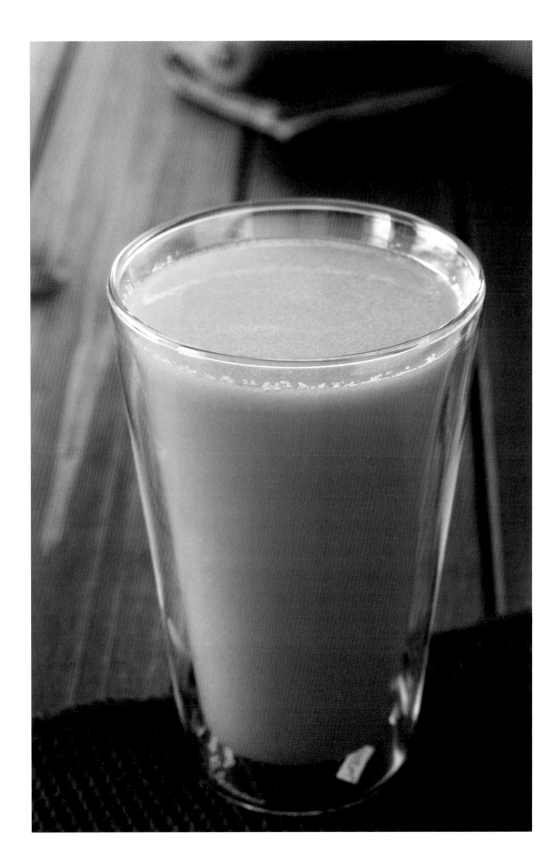

CLEANSE YOUR BODY

A refreshing, intestinal cleansing, and vitalizing drink which steadily improves energy levels

INGREDIENTS

1 cucumber
1 celery stalk
1 piece of ginger (thumbnail-sized)
5 mint leaves
2 stalks of fennel

PREPARATION

Wash and drain all the ingredients, then pat dry using a cloth or paper towel.

Peel the cucumber unless you are using an organic one. Chop everything into pieces small enough to fit through the juicer's filler opening.

Feed the ingredients one by one into the juicer until the juice is ready.

Drink and enjoy immediately!

EFFECT

This is another variation of green juice to help ring the changes. The mint adds more chlorophyll, an excellent blood-cleansing substance, to the classic green juice recipe. Fennel boosts the effect of the drink by adding an extra portion of free-radical interceptors. Both ingredients are excellent both for stimulating the digestive processes and for their calming properties. This juice does not contain fruit or any sweet ingredients and is consequently ideal for anyone with diabetes or candidiasis.

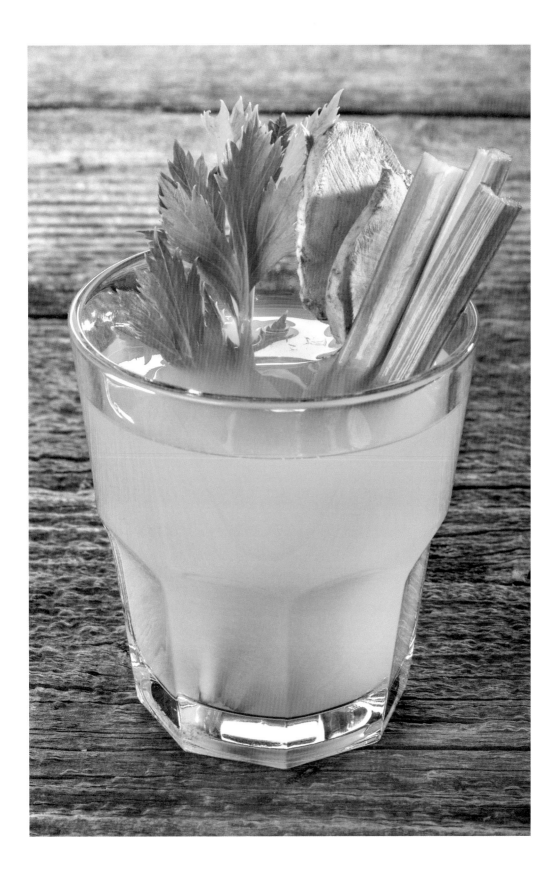

CAPRICHO

*Boosts energy, improves mood, and encourages
a feeling of physical well-being*

INGREDIENTS

1 slice of pineapple
1 beetroot
½ lemon
4 lettuce leaves

PREPARATION

Wash and drain the beetroot and lettuce leaves, then pat dry using a cloth or paper towel. Peel the lemon, then chop everything into pieces small enough to fit through the filler opening of your juicer.

Add the ingredients to the juicer one by one until the juice is ready.

Drink and enjoy immediately!

EFFECT

This juice combines four powerful cleansing ingredients, whilst its sweet flavor makes it a really delicious drink. It cleanses the body in four different ways: beetroot, an excellent ingredient for purifying the blood, stimulates digestion and is good for cleansing the colon. Lemon stimulates the liver and helps to get rid of toxins. Pineapple and lettuce are outstanding natural diuretics and help us to flush any toxins from the body.

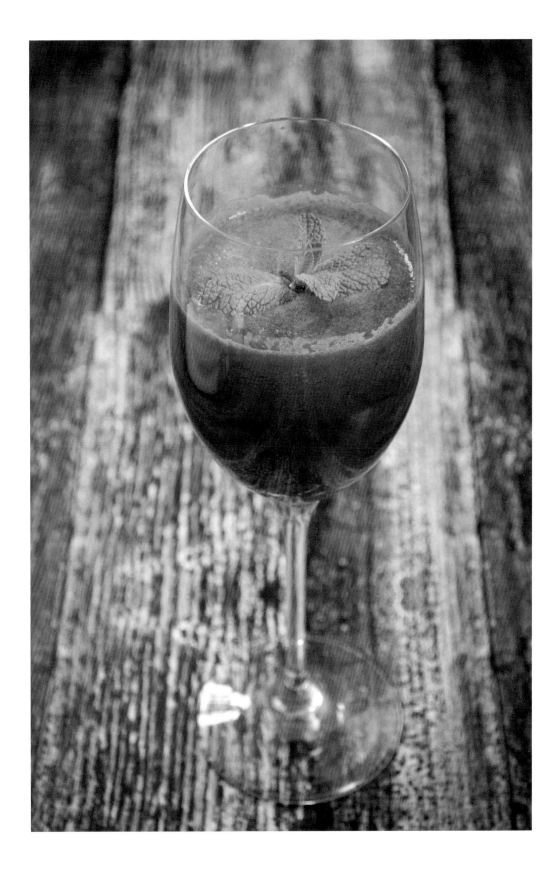

AMOR, AMOR

Energy and pleasure lasting right through the morning!

INGREDIENTS

2 apples
2 beetroots
*1 piece of ginger
    (thumbnail-sized)*

PREPARATION

Wash and drain the three ingredients, then pat dry using a cloth or paper towel. If you are using organic apples, they need not be peeled.

Cut everything into pieces small enough to fit through the filler opening of your juicer.

Feed the ingredients into the juicer one by one. Drink and enjoy immediately!

EFFECT

This juice combines apples and beetroots—two of the most powerful purifying juice ingredients working as a team. In addition to their diuretic properties, which help flush metabolic waste products from the body, it also aids the liver in expelling toxins and has a strong alkalizing effect on the body. This juice will demonstrate how much you love your body and taste buds, its beautiful red color reflecting the passion in your heart.

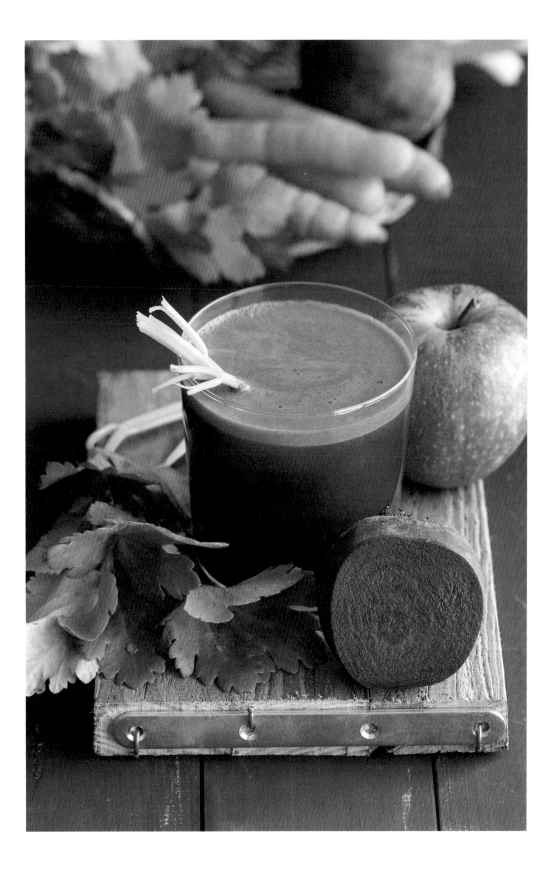

VEGETABLE COCKTAIL

*Restores balance to your body and has a
de-acidifying and detoxifying effect*

INGREDIENTS

2 tomatoes
2 carrots
1 celery stalk
4 sprigs parsley
½ lemon
1 handful of spinach
¼ onion
½ garlic clove (optional)

PREPARATION

Wash and drain all the ingredients except for the lemon, onion, and garlic, then pat dry using a cloth or paper towel. If you are using organic vegetables, there is no need to peel. Otherwise, skin the tomatoes and peel the carrots. Peel the lemon, onion, and garlic also. Cut everything into pieces small enough to fit through the filler opening in your juicer.

Add the ingredients to the juicer one by one until the juice is ready.

Drink and enjoy immediately!

EFFECT

This cocktail is rich in lycopene and antioxidants and tastes very much like gazpacho.

Thanks to its powerful anti-inflammatory, de-acidifying, and detoxifying properties, it is also a useful anti-carcinogenic.

Try it with a topping of turmeric and black pepper to increase its effectiveness.

Garnished with a few celery leaves this cocktail becomes an attractive, refreshing, and healthy aperitif which prepares the stomach for its forthcoming meal.

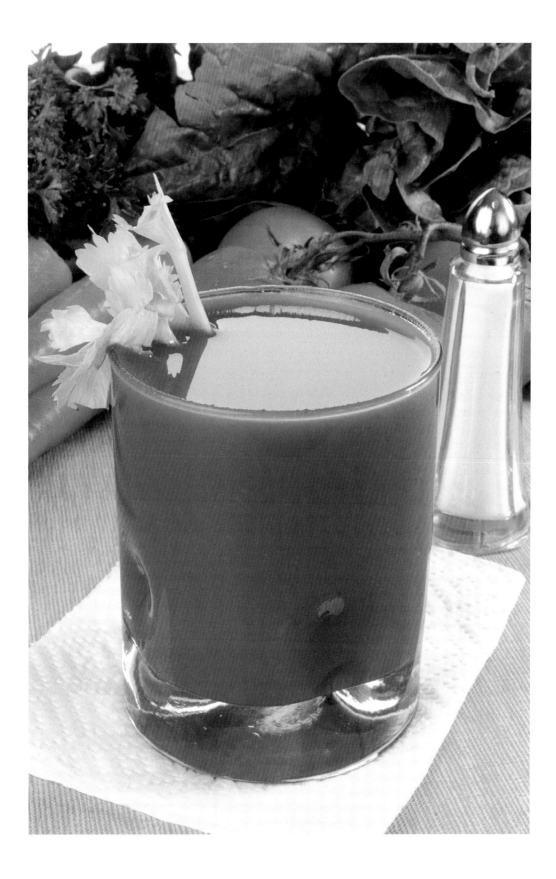

VITAMIN V

· ·

For healthy kidney function

INGREDIENTS

4 sticks of asparagus
3 celery stalks
¼ cabbage
½ apple
1 lemon

PREPARATION

Wash and drain all the ingredients, then pat dry with a cloth or paper towel. If you are using an organic apple, there is no need to peel it.

Peel the lemon. Chop all the ingredients into pieces small enough to fit through the filler opening of your juicer.

Add the ingredients to the juice one after another until the juice is ready.

Drink and enjoy immediately!

EFFECT

If you suffer from fluid retention, want to lose weight, or are prone to infections of the urinary tract, you will find this natural diuretic juice very beneficial.

In addition to its cleansing effect, its diuretic properties help eliminate toxins from the body. This juice is consequently a useful remedy in the treatment of rheumatism, joint disorders, and gout.

It can also improve edematous skin conditions in people suffering from fluid retention.

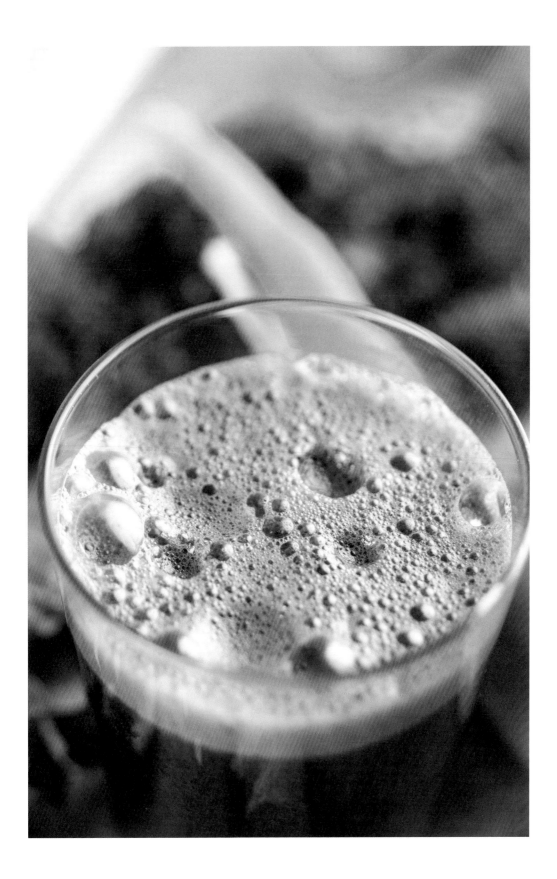

HAPPY LIVER

As the name suggests, this is a great liver cleanser

INGREDIENTS

*2 handfuls of dandelion
   leaves*
*1 handful of alfalfa
   sprouts*
1 cucumber
10 sprigs of parsley
2 lemons
1 green apple

PREPARATION

Wash and drain all the ingredients except for the lemons, then pat dry using a cloth or paper towel. If using organic produce, there is no need to peel the ingredients. Otherwise, peel the cucumber, apple, and lemons. Cut everything into pieces small enough to fit through the filler opening of your juicer.

Add the ingredients to the juicer one by one until the juice is ready.

Drink and enjoy immediately!

EFFECT

The liver's job is to get rid of toxins which have accumulated in the body.

It is also involved in breaking down proteins and cholesterol, which is why it is very important for our health that the liver is functioning properly.

Occasionally, the liver can become so clogged up that it finds it difficult to get rid of waste products. This juice is excellent for supporting the liver in all its functions. Keeping the liver free of an excessive amount of toxins will increase your energy levels and raise your spirits whilst indirectly helping to boost the immune system.

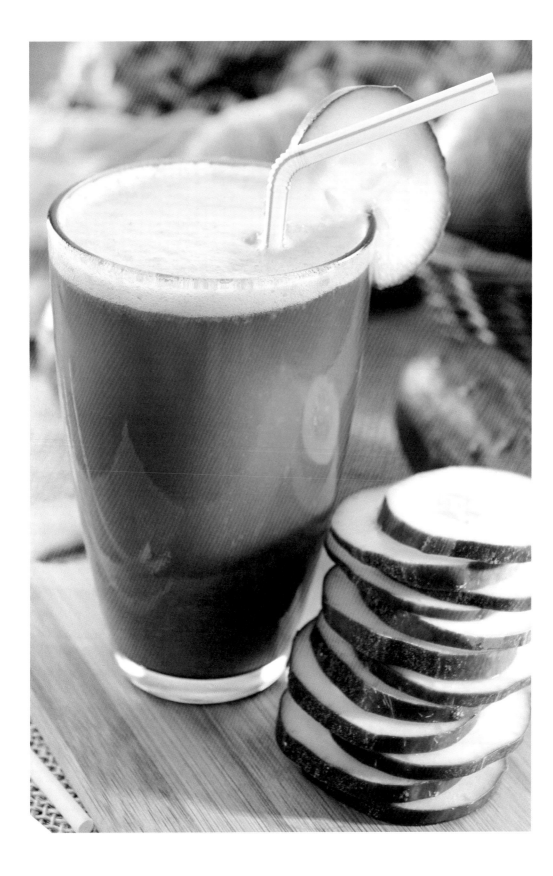

DETOX

*For a serious energy boost
and for regenerating the blood*

INGREDIENTS

1 head of broccoli
5 sprigs of parsley
2 celery stalks
½ cucumber
1 handful of spinach

PREPARATION

Wash and drain all the ingredients, then pat dry with a cloth or paper towel. Peel the cucumber unless it is organic. Cut everything into pieces small enough to fit through the filler opening in your juicer.

Feed the ingredients into the juicer one by one until the juice is ready.

Drink and enjoy immediately!

EFFECT

Chlorophyll has a structure very similar to that of hemoglobin as well as having countless positive effects on our health: it stimulates cell metabolism, detoxifies the body, boosts the body's immune system, supports the natural healing processes, encourages the production of red blood corpuscles, prevents cancer, stops infections, and cleanses the blood. To add an extra portion of chlorophyll to your juice, simply add a topping of one teaspoon of spirulina.

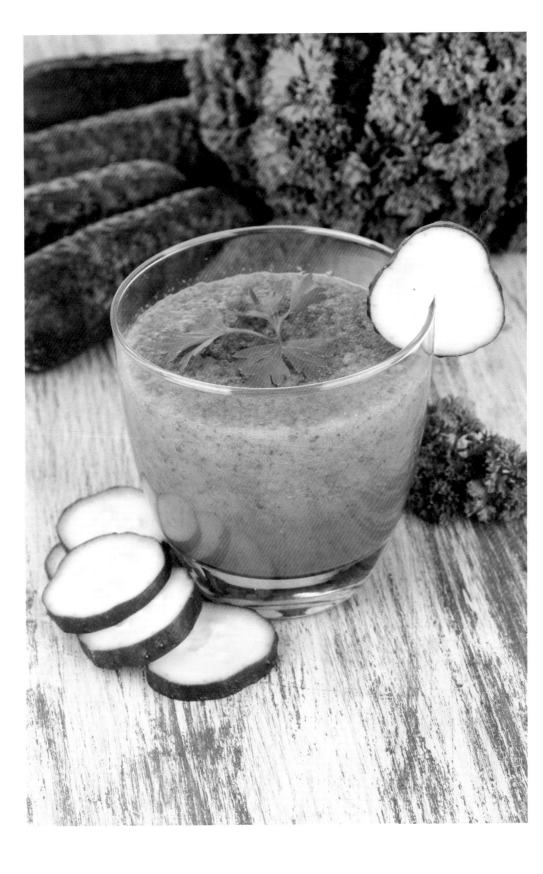

BLOODY GREEN

A vegetable combination which is good for the liver

INGREDIENTS

5 leaves of romaine lettuce
1 cucumber
½ lemon
10 sprigs of parsley

PREPARATION

Wash and drain all the ingredients except for the lemon, then pat dry with a cloth or paper towel. Peel the cucumber unless it is organic. Peel the lemon. Cut everything into pieces small enough to fit through the filler opening of your juicer.

Feed the ingredients into the juicer one by one until the juice is ready.

Drink and enjoy immediately!

EFFECT

Sometimes, when we find ourselves under constant stress, we forget to breathe calmly and evenly. This deprives our body of crucial oxygen. Furthermore, a diet based on excessive amounts of animal protein, saturated fatty acids, and ready meals uses up oxygen in our blood and gradually leads to over-acidification—which can ultimately lead to disease. If consumed on an empty stomach, this juice will help to de-acidify the body.

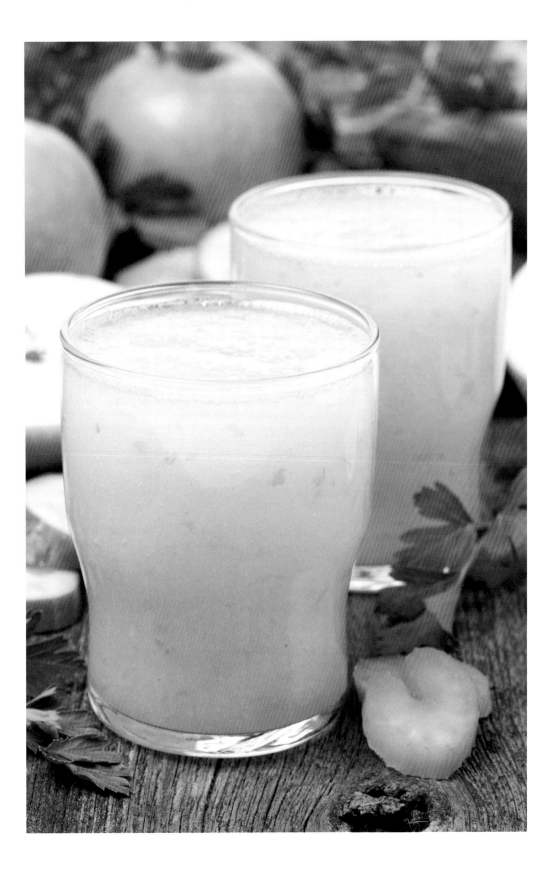

IRON BOOSTER

....

Helps to fight anemia, boost energy,
and promote emotional equilibrium

INGREDIENTS

2 handfuls of spinach
1 beetroot
1 carrot
3 celery stalks
1 lemon

PREPARATION

Wash and drain all the ingredients except for the lemon, then pat dry with a cloth or paper towel. If the carrot is organic, it will not need peeling. Peel the lemon. Cut everything into pieces small enough to fit through the filler opening in your juicer.

Feed the ingredients into the juicer one by one until the juice is ready.

Drink and enjoy immediately!

EFFECT

People considering a high-vegetable diet without any animal protein often worry about a potential lack of iron. However, this need not always be the inevitable consequence of a meat-free diet. Vegetables, grain, and pulses also contain a lot of iron.

This juice drink is a wonderful cocktail of iron and vitamin C, ideal for fighting anemia and stimulating the production of red blood corpuscles. If you want to intensify its effect, you can add a topping of one teaspoon of spirulina.

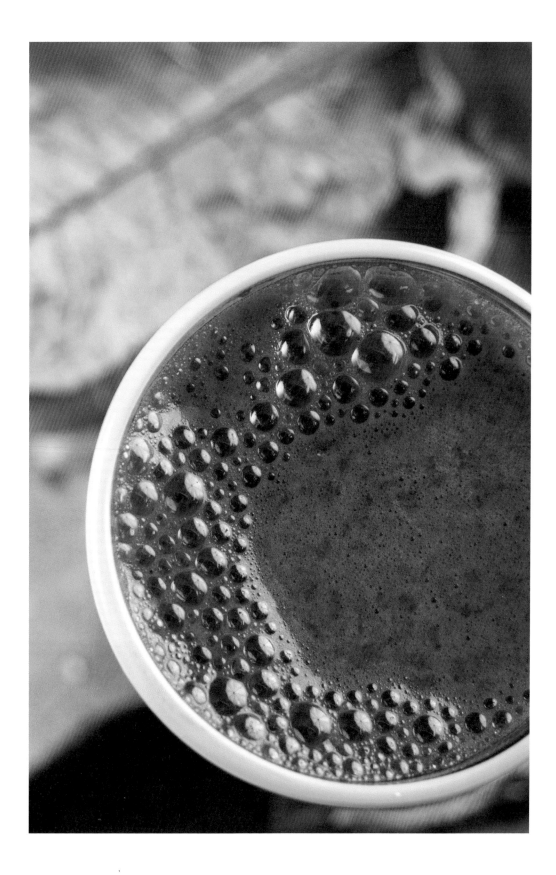

VITAMIN C SPRITZER

....

Rich in vitamin C, boosts the immune system

INGREDIENTS

1 grapefruit
½ lemon
1 cucumber
2 lettuce leaves

PREPARATION

Wash and drain the lettuce leaves, then pat dry using a cloth or paper towel. Peel the grapefruit, lemon, and cucumber. Cut everything into pieces small enough to fit through the filler opening in your juicer.

Feed the ingredients into your juicer one by one until the juice is ready.

Drink and enjoy immediately!

EFFECT

This juice is ideal for increasing our vitamin C reserves. It is highly recommended for weathering the transition of the seasons or when our vitamin C reserves are depleted; it is also useful during periods of stress and during cold weather when we are increasingly susceptible to colds, or if we smoke and take too few breaks.

This juice also makes an ideal hangover cure for the morning after as vitamin C helps to accelerate the breakdown of alcohol. Anemia sufferers are advised to drink the juice 30 minutes before a meal as vitamin C also helps to bind calcium.

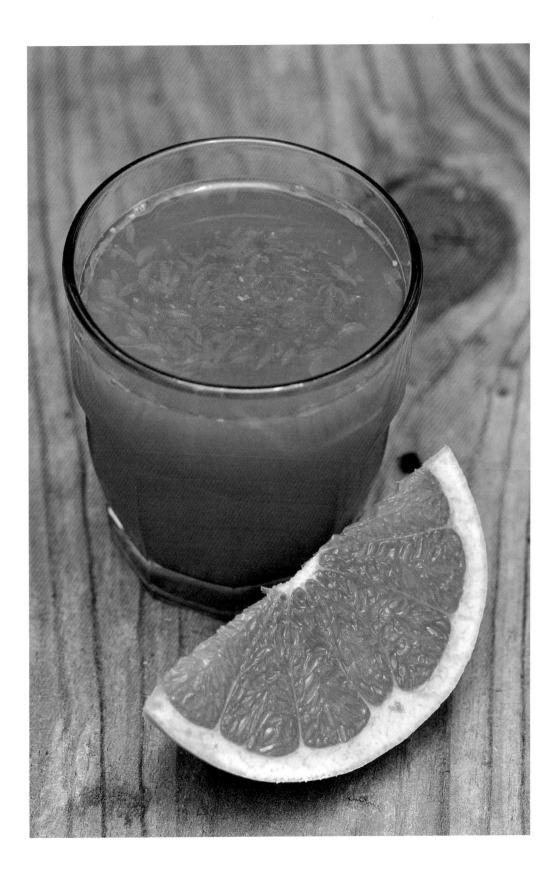

FREEDOM

Maintains healthy iron levels in the blood—and protects against colds and infections

INGREDIENTS

1 carrot
2 oranges
½ cucumber
1 piece of ginger
4 mint leaves
1 tbsp flower pollen

PREPARATION

Wash and drain all the ingredients except for the oranges, then pat dry with a cloth or paper towel. Peel the cucumber and carrot unless they are organic, then peel the oranges. Cut everything into pieces small enough to fit into the filler opening of your juicer.

Feed the ingredients into your juicer one by one.

Drink and enjoy immediately!

EFFECT

This juice is a delicious preventative remedy during the changing seasons when we need to boost our body's defenses. Rich in vitamin C and beta-carotenes, it helps to boost the immune system.

Mint also has anti-viral properties and acts as an expectorant to relieve respiratory-tract congestion. Ginger and flower pollen are excellent natural antibiotics and fight infectious bacteria.

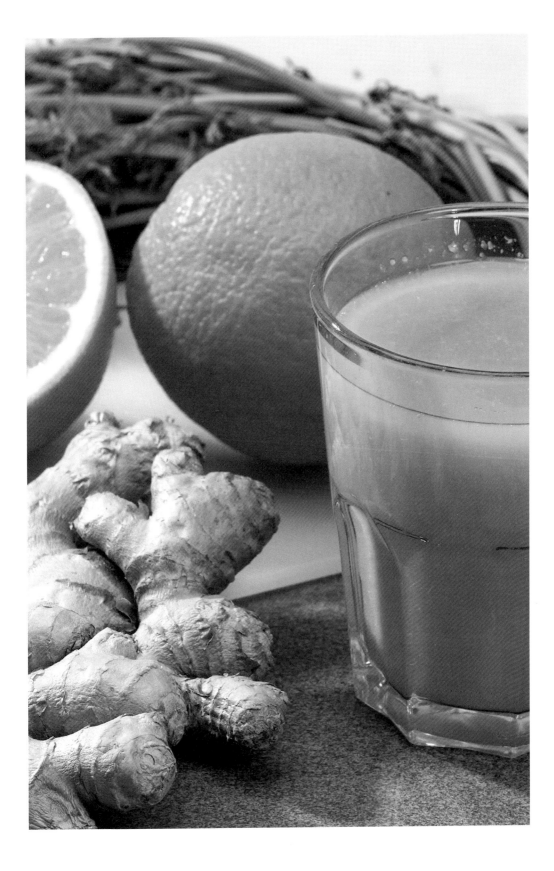

IMMUNE BOOST

. . . .

Better protection from diseases,
allergies, colds, and infections

INGREDIENTS

5 carrots
5 sprigs of parsley
1 handful of spinach
2 celery stalks
1 piece of ginger
  (thumbnail-sized)

PREPARATION

Wash and drain all the ingredients, then pat dry using a cloth or paper towel. Peel the carrots unless they are organic. Cut everything into pieces small enough to fit through the filler opening of your juicer.

Feed the ingredients into the juicer one by one until the juice is ready.

Drink and enjoy immediately!

EFFECT

Our immune system is like an army on stand-by, ready to defend our body against enemies, in other words, diseases of every kind. If the immune system is compromised, it will not be able to defend itself, so that we are more likely to catch a cold or fall prey to more serious illness. It is a good idea, therefore, to boost the immune system regularly by drinking simple juices like this one.

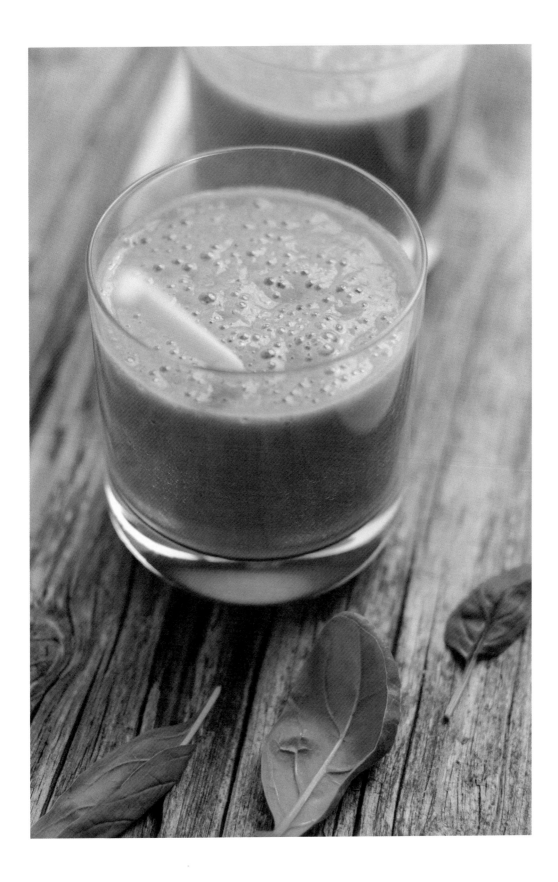

HEALTH CURE

· ·

Acts as an anti-inflammatory, maintains and repairs our cells' inner balance

INGREDIENTS

2 celery stalks

1 cucumber

1 green apple

5 basil leaves

1 piece of ginger (thumbnail-sized)

1 piece of turmeric root (thumbnail-sized)

PREPARATION

Wash and drain all the ingredients, then pat dry with a cloth or paper towel. If you are using organic produce, it will not need peeling. Otherwise peel the apple and cucumber. Cut everything into pieces small enough to fit through your juicer's filler opening.

Feed the ingredients into the juicer one by one until the juice is ready.

Drink and enjoy immediately!

EFFECT

Highly recommended to maintain the function of the body's organs and tissue. Whenever inflammation occurs in the body, toxins are produced, which can lead to the development of disease. Any ailments which ended in "-itis" indicate an inflammation which upsets the balance of our well-being. Ongoing or chronic inflammation conditions can lead to serious illnesses such as cancer, Alzheimer's, or arterial sclerosis. This "health cure" juice contains concentrated levels of anti-inflammatory and cleansing plant-based substances, which help to prevent and fight such inflammation.

GREEN JUICE RECIPES—FOR BOOSTING THE IMMUNE SYSTEM

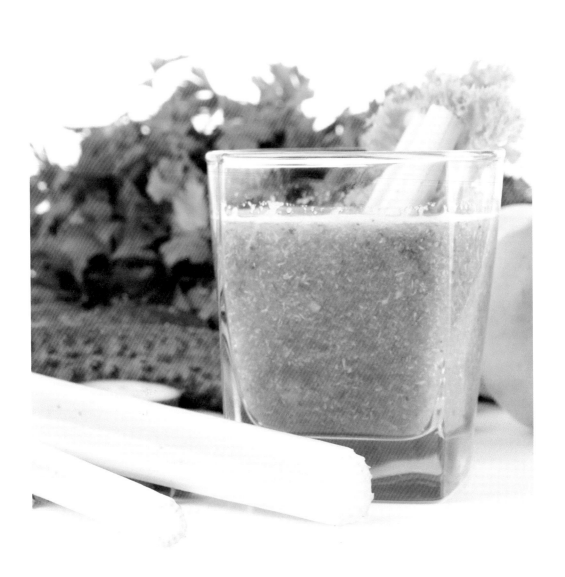

ENERGY POWER

....

Restores physical and emotional balance
and creates a feeling of well-being

INGREDIENTS

15 red grapes
2 celery stalks
½ cucumber
½ lime
1 handful of basil

PREPARATION

Wash and drain all the ingredients except for the lime, then pat dry using a cloth or paper towel. Peel the cucumber unless it is an organic one. Peel the lime. Cut everything into pieces small enough to fit through the filler opening of your juicer.

Feed the ingredients into the juicer one by one until the juice is ready.

Drink and enjoy immediately!

EFFECT

This regenerating juice is ideal for athletes, students, or people in convalescence. Red grapes are an excellent natural source of energy. At the same time, the cleansing and anti-oxidative effect of this juice helps to eliminate free radicals and metabolic waste products resulting from the extra physical demands placed on people in the above-mentioned groups. Basil also helps to strengthen and stabilize the nervous system. Grapes, because of their sugar content, are not suitable for diabetics.

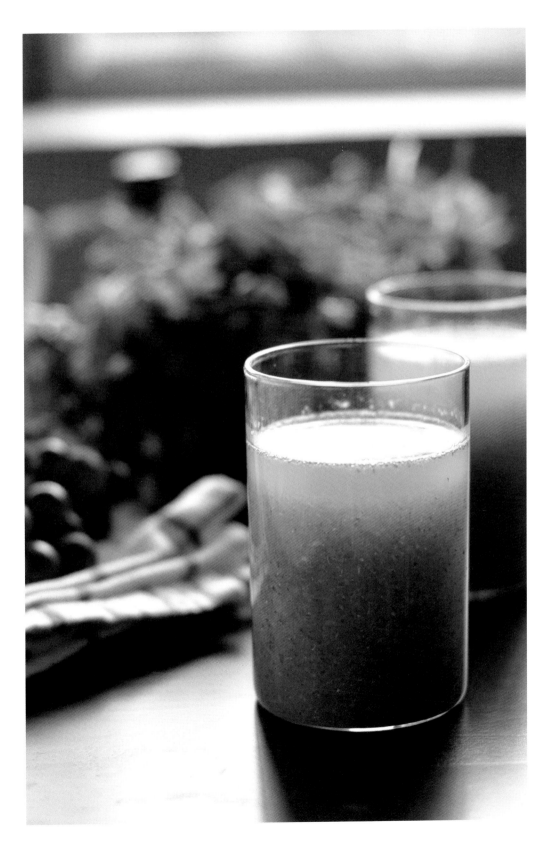

SWEET WAKE-UP

Increases vitality, energy, and powers of concentration

INGREDIENTS

1 apple
1 pear
1 grapefruit
2 celery stalks
1 piece of ginger
  (thumbnail-sized)

PREPARATION

Wash and drain all the ingredients except for the grapefruit, then pat dry with a cloth or paper towel. Organic produce does not need peeling. Peel the grapefruit.

Cut everything into pieces small enough to fit through the filler opening of your juicer.

Feed the ingredients into the juicer one by one until the juice is ready.

Drink and enjoy immediately!

EFFECT

This juice can replace your morning coffee as its high fruit content will provide a powerful boost of good energy. The energy kick provided by coffee is deceptive because it demands a quid pro quo: its absorption actually uses up energy and depletes the body's nutrient reserves. This is why one cup of coffee is often not enough. Regular coffee drinkers will undoubtedly have already noticed this vicious circle. Juices, on the other hand, simply give but take nothing in return: vitamins, minerals, enzymes, fibers, trace elements, electrolytes … all substances which supply high concentrations of energy.

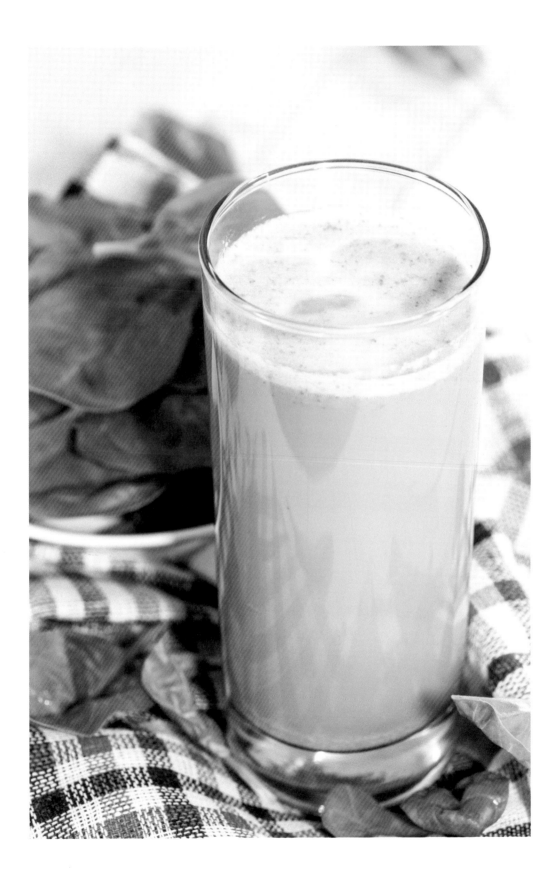

RAINBOW

An anti-aging juice for younger, firmer, hydrated, and glowing skin

INGREDIENTS

½ red or yellow bell pepper
* (whichever you prefer)*
1 beetroot
4 carrots
6 leaves of romaine lettuce
1 cucumber

PREPARATION

Wash and drain all the ingredients, then pat dry with a cloth or paper towel. If the carrots and cucumber are organic, they do not need peeling. Cut everything into pieces small enough to fit through the filler opening of your juicer.

Feed the ingredients into the juicer one by one until the juice is ready.

Drink and enjoy immediately!

EFFECT

This green juice recipe creates a rainbow-colored glass of juice. It contains a perfect balance of vitamin C and beta-carotene, two antioxidants which are vital for keeping skin young and beautiful.

Cucumber regenerates and hydrates the cells and improves vitality. If we include red bell pepper, the juice will also provide us with lycopene, another substance which plays a significant role in slowing down our cells' aging process.

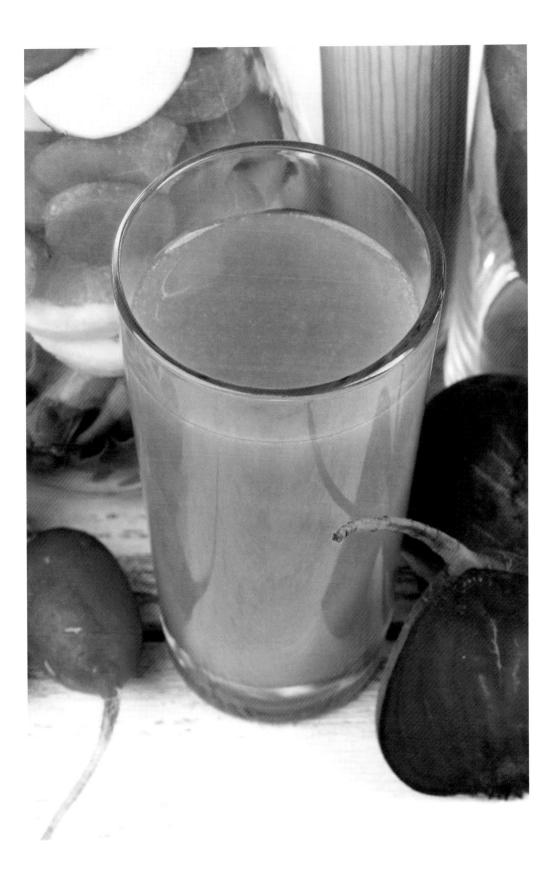

VISION BOOSTER

· ·

Improves vision and promotes summer tanning

INGREDIENTS

1 apple
5 carrots
2 handfuls of spinach
1 piece of ginger (optional)

PREPARATION

Wash and drain all the ingredients, then pat dry with a cloth or paper towel. If the carrots and apple are organic, they do not need peeling. Cut everything into pieces small enough to fit through the filler opening of your juicer.

Feed the ingredients one by one into the juicer until the juice is ready.

Drink and enjoy immediately!

EFFECT

Drinking this juice will not only enhance your appearance but also improve your vision. Its high content of beta-carotenes (precursors of vitamin A), which inhibit cell damage, make this juice a powerful antioxidant, improving not only the health of your skin but your vision as well. It is good for alleviating night blindness and hypersensitivity to sunlight, and preventing cataracts.

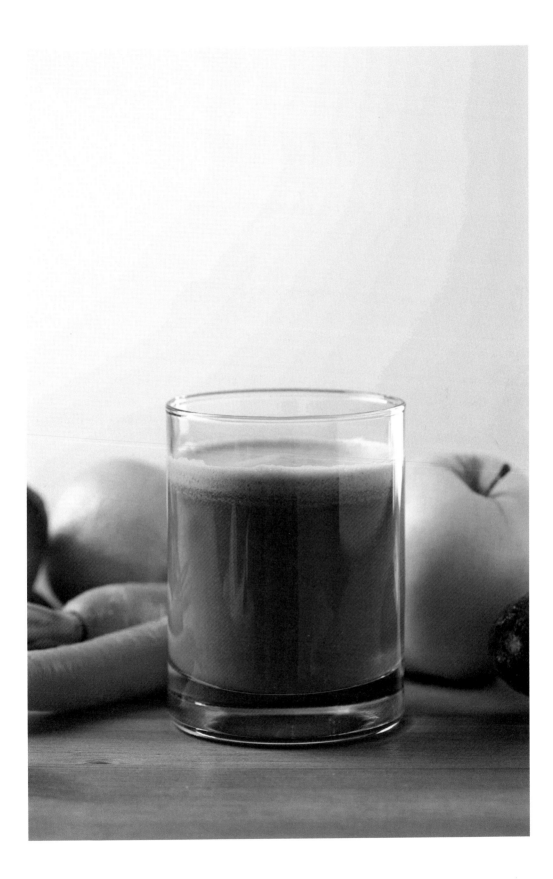

TROPICAL

....

Has a detoxifying effect which also reduces cellulite

INGREDIENTS

2 slices of pineapple
½ cucumber
2 celery stalks
2 handfuls of spinach

PREPARATION

Wash and drain all the ingredients except for the pineapple, then pat dry using a cloth or paper towel. If the cucumber is organic, it will not need peeling. Cut everything into pieces small enough to fit through the opening of your juicer.

Feed the ingredients one by one into the juicer until the juice is ready.

Drink and enjoy immediately!

EFFECT

This powerful diuretic cocktail counteracts water retention. The star ingredient in this respect is pineapple, which contains bromelain, a substance with anti-inflammatory and diuretic properties. It also relieves edematous conditions connected with cellulite.

Drinking this rather exotic-flavored juice on a daily basis on an empty stomach, combined with a little exercise and a healthy diet with lots of vegetables, but no sugar or saturated fatty acids, will help tackle cellulite.

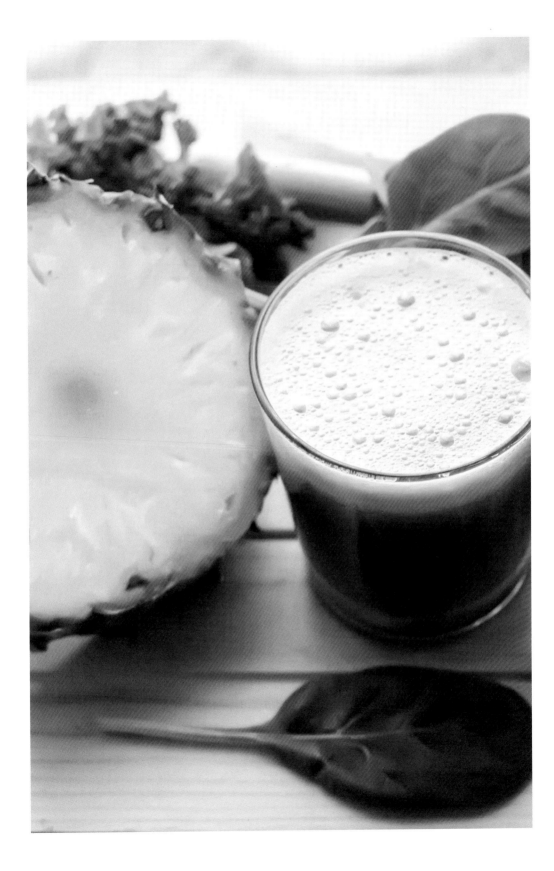

ANTI-AGING

*An antioxidant—promoting soft, radiant skin,
and a healthy appearance*

INGREDIENTS

1 grapefruit
6 carrots
1 handful of spinach
*1 piece of ginger
(thumbnail-sized)*

PREPARATION

Wash and drain all the ingredients except for the grapefruit, then pat dry using a cloth or paper towel. If the carrots are organic, they will not need peeling. Peel the grapefruit. Cut everything into pieces small enough to fit through the filler opening of your juicer.

Feed in the ingredients one by one until the juice is ready.

Drink and enjoy immediately!

EFFECT

If you are looking for a juice to give you beautiful skin, you should select ingredients which are rich in vitamin C and beta-carotenes. In which case, this is the perfect drink for you, and its impact is heightened by the iron content in spinach. Iron is crucial for transporting oxygen to body tissue; the vitamin C content in the juice also supports the body's ability to absorb iron. Whereas people with anemia tend to be rather pale, adequate iron levels in the blood will guarantee a healthy complexion.

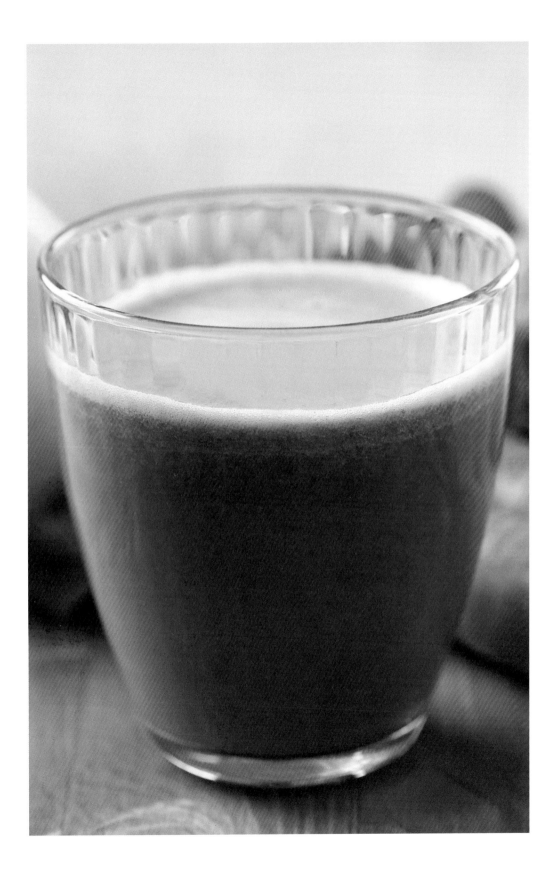

DELI

Helps contribute to a radiant complexion—and takes a few years off your age

INGREDIENTS

4 carrots
2 Granny Smith apples
1 beetroot

PREPARATION

Wash and drain all three ingredients, then pat dry using a cloth or paper towel. If you are using organic fruit and vegetables, they will not need peeling. Cut everything into pieces small enough to fit through the filler opening of your juicer.

Feed the ingredients into the juicer one by one until the juice is ready.

Drink and enjoy immediately!

EFFECT

The advantage of this juice is that, despite only consisting of a few ingredients, it has high levels of antioxidants in the form of vitamin C and beta-carotenes.

Thanks to the beetroot, this juice is also rich in folic acid, which is essential for generating new tissue. Its cleansing properties also help promote radiant skin. And the best thing about this juice is its delicious, sweet flavor.

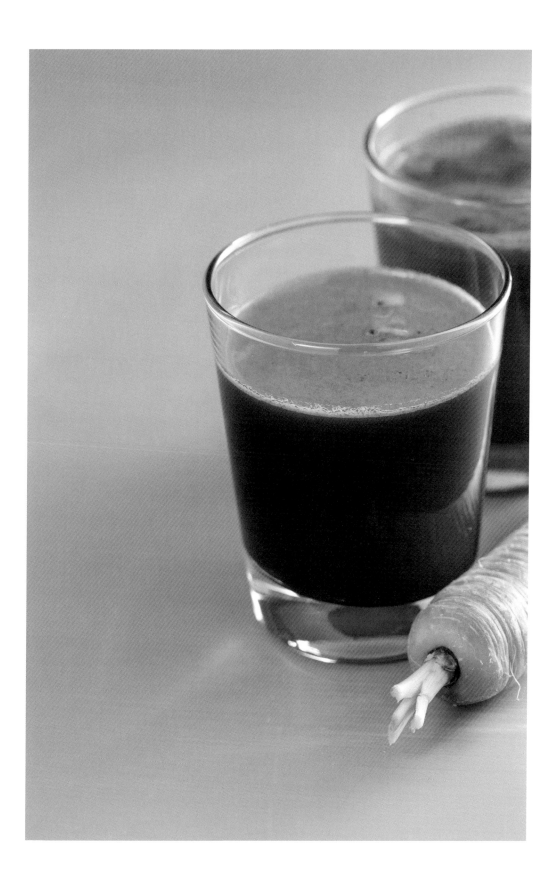

SUNSHINE

···

For young-looking skin with fewer wrinkles

INGREDIENTS

1 red bell pepper
2 carrots
1 apple
1 piece of ginger
  (thumbnail-sized)
1 tbsp hemp seeds

PREPARATION

Wash and drain all the ingredients, then pat dry using a cloth or paper towels. If the apples and carrots are organic, they will not need peeling.

Cut everything into pieces small enough to fit through filler opening of your juicer.

Feed the ingredients into the juicer one by one until the juice is ready.

Drink and enjoy immediately!

EFFECT

This sweet juice with its zingy flavor boasts almost magical properties consisting as it does of all the ingredients necessary to promote eternal youth: vitamins A, C, D, and E, lycopene, polyphenols, and omega 3 fatty acids.

The hemp seeds in this juice are essential as they supply vitamin E and omega 3 fatty acids. If you drink this juice every day, you will literally be able to see the hands of time moving backwards.

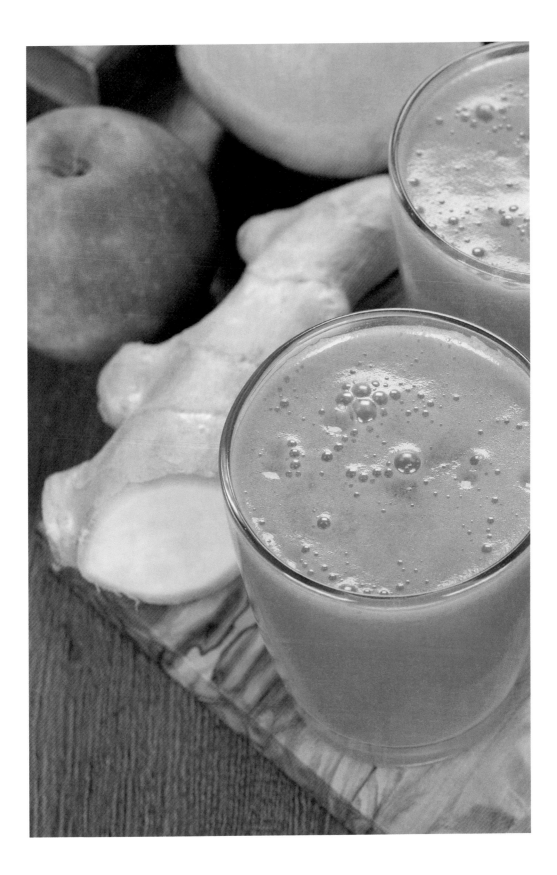

FLAT BELLY

*Absorbs stomach acid and helps promote
well-being*

INGREDIENTS

½ cabbage
5 carrots
2 celery stalks
½ cucumber

PREPARATION

Wash and drain all the ingredients and pat dry using a cloth or paper towel. If the carrots and cucumber are organic, they will not need peeling. Cut everything into pieces small enough to fit through the filler opening in your juicer.

Feed the ingredients one by one into the juicer until the juice is ready.

Drink and enjoy immediately!

EFFECT

This elixir for the stomach consists of vegetables which are excellent for caring for the stomach lining. Cabbage juice is a natural de-acidifier and increases the production of mucins, a mucous gel which soothes the intestinal passage, acts as a lubricant, and protects the stomach. Cabbage has also been found to help heal injuries to the stomach wall. Celery likewise strengthens the stomach lining and protects the stomach walls.

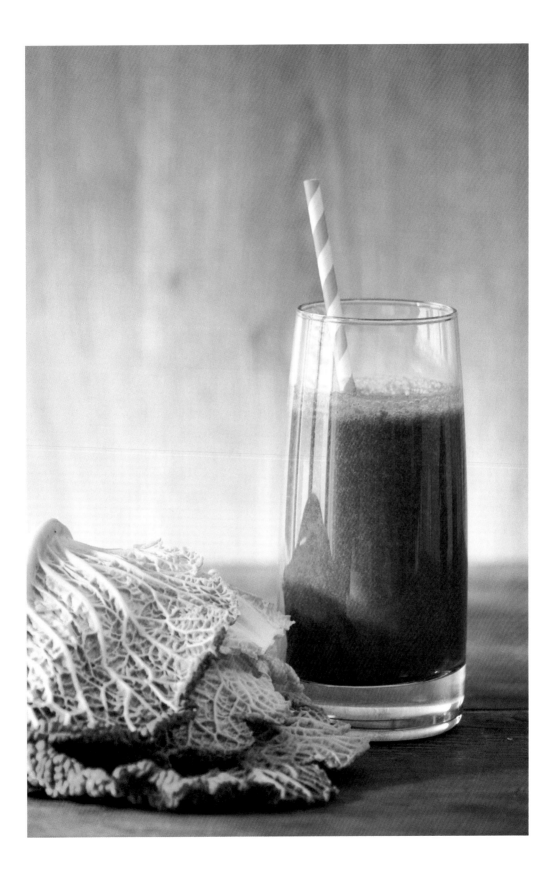

HAPPY DAY

···

*Reduces stomach acid, improves digestion,
and promotes a healthy digestive system*

INGREDIENTS

¼ red cabbage
3 celery stalks
½ lemon
1 apple

PREPARATION

Wash and drain all the ingredients, then pat dry using a cloth or paper towel. If the apple is organic, it will not need peeling. Peel the lemon. Cut everything into pieces small enough to fit through the filler opening of your juicer.

Feed the ingredients one by one into the juicer until the juice is ready.

Drink and enjoy immediately!

EFFECT

One of the main problems we face in our everyday lives is stress, which also has an impact on our physical well-being. The most common adverse effects include stomach hyperacidity, which is unfortunately a very common complaint. This juice, consumed on an empty stomach, is a great way to treat this complaint. It can also be enjoyed a good half-hour before eating to prepare the stomach for its forthcoming meal.

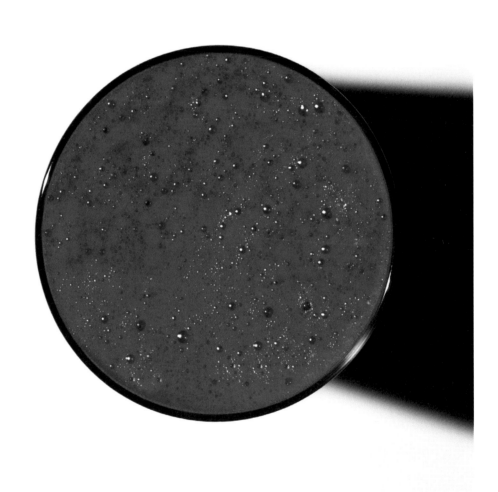

KIWI EXPRESS

....

Aids healthy daily bowel motion—regular as clockwork

INGREDIENTS

2 kiwis
1 apple
2 handfuls of spinach
½ lemon

PREPARATION

Wash and drain the spinach and apple, then pat dry with a cloth or paper towel. Peel the lemon and the kiwi fruit. Cut everything into pieces small enough to fit through the filler hole of your juicer.

Feed the ingredients one by one into the juicer until the juice is ready.

Drink and enjoy immediately!

EFFECT

The purifying effects of this juice are due to the kiwi fruit, which contain magnesium as well as soluble and insoluble fiber. Kiwi, spinach, and apple pectins make a powerful trio of fibers, which prevent constipation and ease bowel motion. If you want to intensify the effects of the juice, you can add Chia seeds. The mucous formed by the seeds in conjunction with fluid makes them swell up and stimulates bowel movement.

Fewer toxins in our body will give us greater mental clarity and increased powers of concentration.

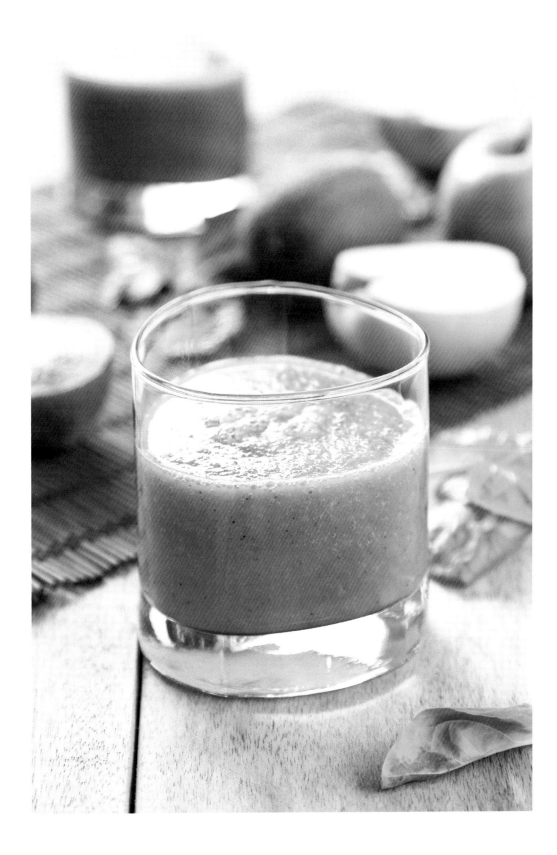

COOL SUMMER

· ·

Leaves you feeling replete and refreshed in the summer heat

INGREDIENTS

¼ watermelon
4 mint leaves
½ lemon

PREPARATION

Wash and drain the mint, then pat dry with a cloth or paper towel. Slice and peel the watermelon and lemon.

Cut everything into pieces small enough to fit through the filler hole of your juicer.

Feed the ingredients one by one into the juicer until the juice is ready.

Drink and enjoy immediately!

EFFECT

Watermelon is one of the most popular summer fruits. The fresh, sweet, juicy flesh is filling and also slakes the thirst. It is rich in citrulline, an amino acid which expands the blood vessels. Combined with the refreshing mint, it turns the juice into a real summer elixir which stimulates and cools down the circulatory system. Impress your guests as the coolest juice expert of the summer!

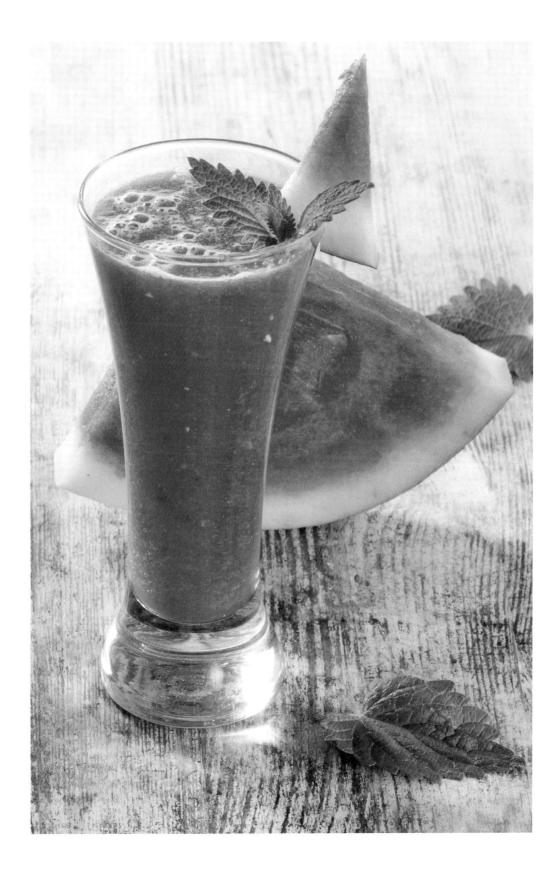

BALANCE

Boosts energy—and helps bring weight under control

INGREDIENTS

6 carrots

1 cucumber

½ lemon

10 radishes

PREPARATION

Wash and drain all the ingredients except for the lemon, then pat dry using a cloth or paper towel. Peel the lemon. If you are using an organic cucumber, this will not need peeling. Cut everything into pieces small enough to fit through the filler opening of your juicer.

Feed the ingredients one by one into the juicer until the juice is ready.

Drink and enjoy immediately!

EFFECT

Thanks to the large quantity of radishes, this surprising juice has the ability to inhibit excess hormone production in the thyroid, thereby helping to stabilize thyroid function. The cucumber contains B-group vitamins, which are likewise essential for healthy thyroid function, especially in the case of hyperactivity. This juice is not particularly recommended for people with an underactive thyroid.

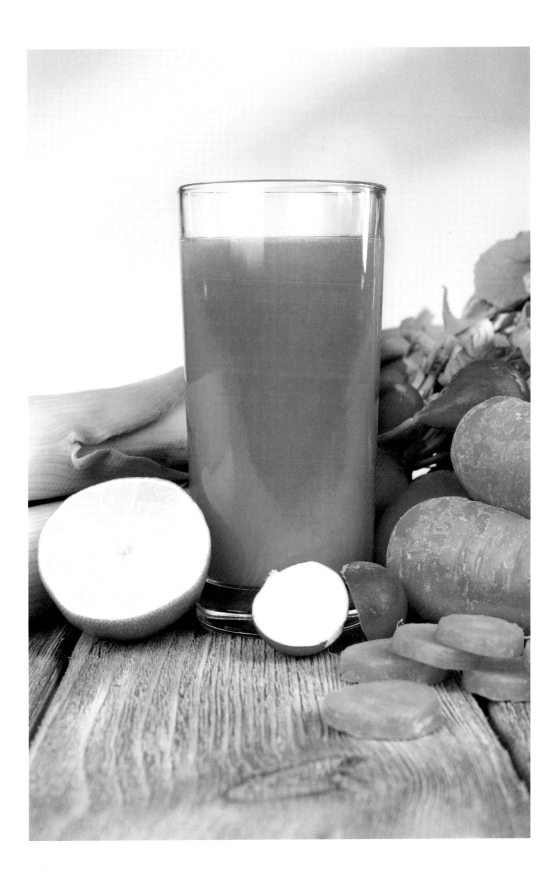

FLOWER POWER

··

Promotes relaxation and equilibrium,
improves powers of concentration and well-being

INGREDIENTS

½ grapefruit
2 celery stalks
½ cucumber
1 garlic clove (optional)
¼ fennel bulb

PREPARATION

Wash all the ingredients except for the grapefruit, then pat dry using a cloth or paper towel. Cut up and peel the grapefruit. If you are using an organic cucumber, it will not need peeling. Cut everything into pieces small enough to fit through the filler hole of your juicer.

Feed the ingredients one by one into the juicer until the juice is ready.

Drink and enjoy immediately!

EFFECT

Stress can arise as a result of changes, tension, or fear. If the stress lasts for any length of time, it will ultimately have a negative impact on our bodies. Certain foods act as anti-stress agents, helping to calm the nervous system, lower blood pressure, and fight stress symptoms such as exhaustion, dehydration, or hyperacidity of the blood. This juice contains some of these anti-stress ingredients.

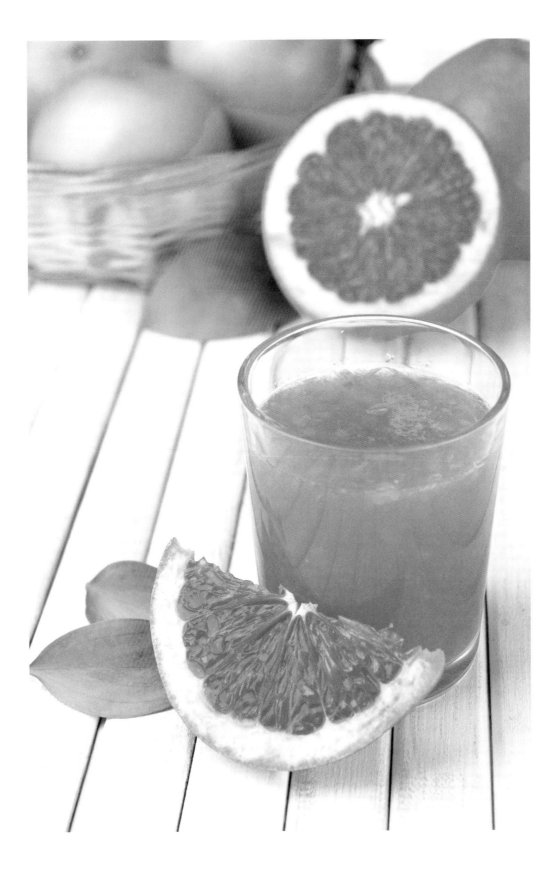

STRONG BONES

∙∙

Helps to keep bones strong and firm for longer

INGREDIENTS

1 head of broccoli
5 sprigs of parsley
3 carrots
1 Granny Smith apple
1 lemon

PREPARATION

Wash and drain all the ingredients, then pat dry using a cloth or paper towel. Peel the lemon. If you are using organic carrots, they will not need peeling.

Cut everything into pieces small enough to fit through the filler opening of your juicer.

Feed the ingredients one by one into the juicer until the juice is ready.

Drink and enjoy immediately!

EFFECT

This juice is perfect for supplying our bones with the optimum amount of calcium. In addition to the calcium in the broccoli and parsley, it also contains other substances which are very important for aiding calcium uptake. These are mainly vitamin D and magnesium, as well as other contributory factors which stimulate absorption, such as vitamins A and C.

Vitamin D is produced from sunlight. If this is in short supply, the chlorophyll molecules in this juice also contain magnesium, which improves calcium absorption. In other words, the chlorophyll acts as a kind of "sunlight storer," regulating calcium levels and balancing out any vitamin D shortfall.

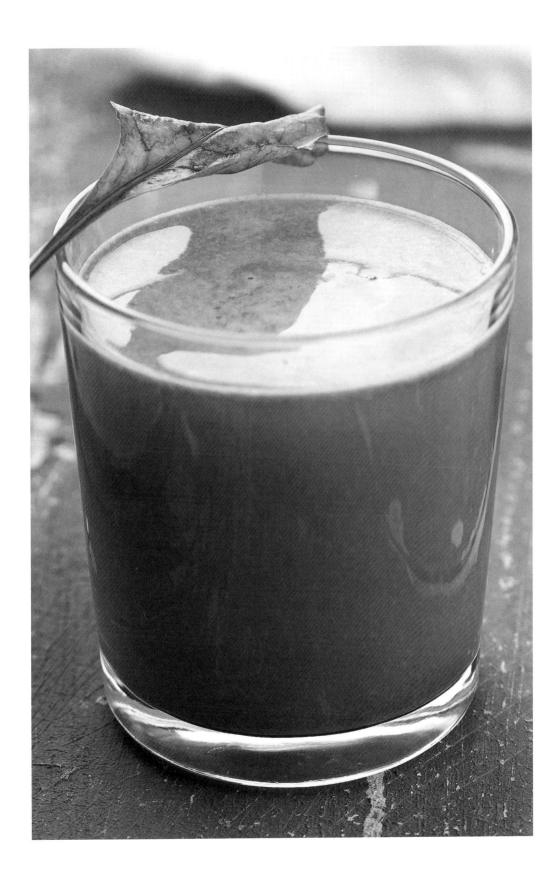

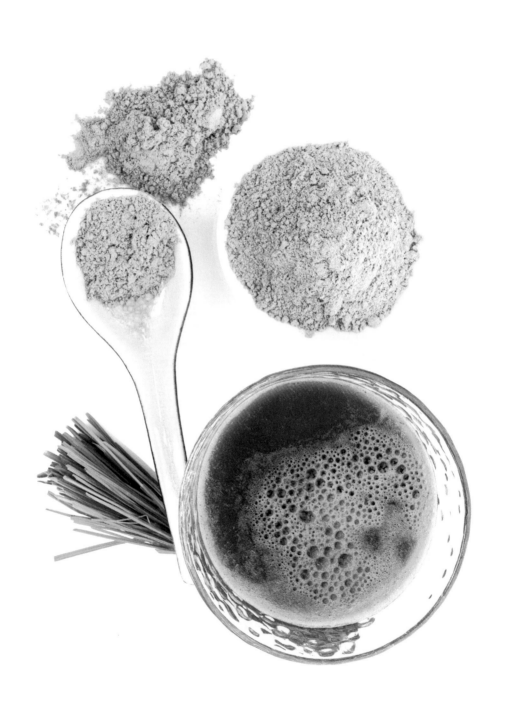

TOPPINGS

Would you like to add a little extra kick to your juices? I would like to devote the final part of my book to introducing you to some of my favorite and most frequently recommended toppings—in other words, additional ingredients you can add to the drinks or sprinkle on top. They are all classed as superfoods— that is to say, ingredients with a high nutrient content which help boost the positive effects of these juices even more.

ACAI BERRIES

They contain up to five times more antioxidants than blueberries

Acai berries come from a type of palm tree native to the tropical and sub-tropical regions of South America. The fruit contains one of the highest concentrations of antioxidants found anywhere in the plant world.

It also acts as a powerful detoxifier and boosts the immune system. It increases the libido, strengthens the nervous system, and also contains large amounts of the essential fatty acids omega 3, 6, and 9, which help to relieve disorders of the heart and circulatory system.

Acai berries are rich in calcium, fiber, vitamins A, E, C, and B vitamins. Most importantly, they contain large amounts of calcium and magnesium as well as significant levels of iron, zinc, and potassium.

ALFALFA SPROUTS

They contain twice as many proteins, four times as much calcium, and twice as much iron as most other vegetables

During germination, alfalfa—like all other grain and vegetable seeds—produce large amounts of nutrients and enzymes, one of the most important being chlorophyll, an important blood cleanser.

Alfalfa sprouts contain diuretic and anti-inflammatory properties. They boost the immune system and keep the nervous system and bones healthy. They also regulate the digestive processes and relieve constipation.

They have a high content of vitamin C, B vitamins, vitamin A, and vitamin K, which plays an essential role in binding calcium and blood-clotting. Alfalfa sprouts are rich in iron and calcium, containing higher levels of these minerals than milk. They also supply phosphorus, magnesium, potassium, and selenium.

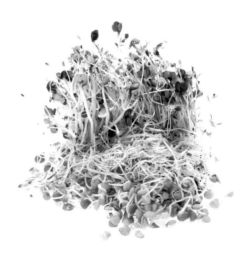

CACAO NIBS OR CACAO POWDER

This valuable superfood is very rich in antioxidants and is therefore excellent for fighting the aging process. It is primarily a good source of magnesium, a mineral which is essential for binding calcium to our bones. It is also useful in treating pre-menstrual syndrome.

Cacao also stimulates the release of endorphins, which promote a feeling of well-being. Rich in polyphenols, it also protects our heart and circulatory system, lowers blood pressure, and helps to prevent blood clots forming.

Although it is good to drink cacao every day, it should not be drunk to excess as its theobromine content can have a similar effect to caffeine.

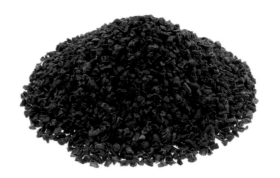

TURMERIC

The best anti-cancer agent

Turmeric is a root. Because of its powerful anti-inflammatory properties, it is highly recommended for relieving pain caused by rheumatism or arthritis.

It also helps to alleviate inflammation in the mouth (if the powder is used as a mouth wash). Sensitive gums can also be treated by sprinkling a little turmeric powder onto your toothbrush.

Turmeric also protects the liver and is a good detoxifier. It helps to prevent blood clots from forming as it stops thrombocytes from clumping together, thereby improving circulation and preventing arterial sclerosis.

Turmeric contains ten anti-oxidative substances. It has been shown to be very valuable as an anti-carcinogenic in three different ways:

It helps fight cancerous substances, boosts the body's own production of anti-carcinogenic substances, and regulates the various factors which can lead to the growth of tumors.

These anti-carcinogenic properties are augmented if combined with another spice: black pepper.

Turmeric improves digestion and helps prevent intestinal gases.

It contains vitamin C, vitamin B3, iron, zinc, selenium, and manganese.

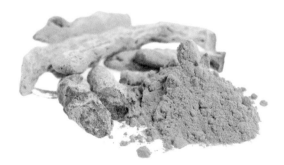

SPIRULINA

This alga gets its blue-green color from its high chlorophyll content, which makes it an excellent blood detoxifier. Spirulina was awarded superfood status by the United Nations for treating anemia and malnutrition in humanitarian emergencies. It contains proteins and iron, which are more easily digestible and absorbable than those contained in meat. Thanks to its numerous antioxidants, it is an excellent anti-aging agent and replenishes energy reserves after sport or exercise or in the case of exhaustion, hence its importance for athletes.

It contains fourteen times as much iron as meat. Its main minerals are beta-carotene and linoleic acid. Spirulina is rich in vitamin E, calcium, phosphorus, and magnesium. It contains essential fatty acids which are not present in meat, fish, or eggs.

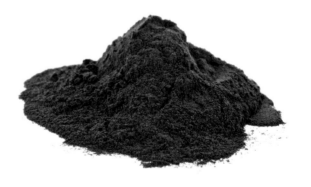

WHEAT GRASS

Alkalizes like no other ingredient

Wheat grass is a star topping for any green juice. It is one of the most efficient of all alkalizing agents and regulates the blood's pH value. It contains large amounts of chlorophyll and consequently plays a very important role in cell renewal, detoxification, and strengthening the circulatory system.

Wheat grass also cleanses the digestive system. Studies carried out by Ann Wigmore (founder of the Hippocrates Health Institute in the USA) have shown that it can be helpful in fighting cancer and other serious illnesses such as diabetes. It not only rids the body of toxins but also eliminates heavy metals whilst detoxing the liver.

Wheat grass contains high concentrations of vitamin A and vitamin C as well as minerals such as calcium, potassium, zinc, magnesium, and iron.

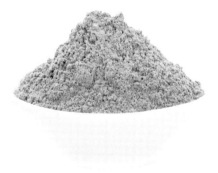

MACA ROOT

Mental and physical super power

Maca is outstanding for boosting vitality and increasing the body's physical and mental resistance capacity, which is why it is especially good for athletes or for children and adults who are weakened by illness. It also strengthens and regulates the hormone system, alleviates symptoms connected with the menopause, and stabilizes the menstrual cycle. It increases fertility, heightens the libido, and improves sexual function. Its high levels of iron relieve the symptoms of anemia.

In addition to all the essential amino acids, it also contains large amounts of vitamins B1, B2, C, and E as well as minerals such as calcium, potassium, phosphorus, iodine, and magnesium.

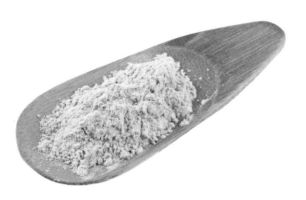

FLOWER POLLEN

Flower pollen is loaded with nutrients and a natural energizer which simultaneously boosts the immune system, particularly during the change of seasons. Not only does it have anti-bacterial properties, but it also stabilizes the blood's pH value and increases hemoglobin levels, thereby helping to regenerate the blood.

Flower pollen is a powerful nutrient which, if consumed regularly, can be a universal remedy for a wide range of problems: menstruation- or menopause-related problems, constipation, diarrhea, anxiety, depression, anemia, convalescence, chronic fatigue, digestive complaints, rheumatism, tissue inflammation, colds, weakness aggravated by seasonal change.

It contains a large number of enzymes and vitamins (all the B-group vitamins as well as vitamins A, D, E, and C), in addition to minerals or oligo-elements such as calcium, chlorine, copper, iron, magnesium, manganese, phosphorus, potassium, silicon, sulfur, and antibiotic substances.

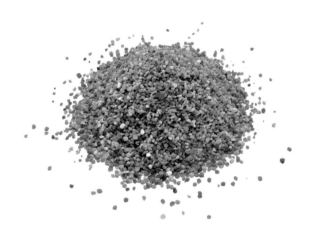

HEMP SEEDS

Good source of plant protein

Contrary to what one might expect, hemp seeds do not contain any psycho-active substances but are instead an excellent source of plant proteins which are easily absorbed, digestible, and bioavailable since they contain all the essential amino acids and, unlike soya, do not come from GM cultivation. Thanks to their high concentration of omega 3 and omega 6 fatty acids, they are highly recommended in the prevention or treatment of heart and circulatory disorders. They are also useful for maintaining a healthy immune system as well as being a powerful antioxidant.

They contain a large number of vitamins: A, C, D, B, and E. The main minerals in hemp seed are calcium, phosphorus, and iron—three minerals which are essential for sound tissue and a strong bone structure.

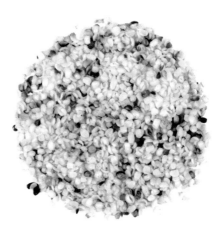

CHIA SEEDS

Seven times more omega 3 fatty acids than salmon

Chia seeds are reputed to contain twice as much protein as any other seeds and five times as much calcium as milk. They also contain large amounts of omega 3 fatty acid, more than salmon or linseed. Since the seeds absorb ten times their weight in water and consequently develop into a thick gel, they reduce appetite and produce a feeling of fullness. They also prevent blood-sugar levels from rising, which is why they are very useful for diabetes sufferers.

Chia seeds are also rich in antioxidants. They strengthen the immune system and have anti-carcinogenic properties.

They also supply vitamin C and B-group vitamins, especially vitamin B3. The main minerals include potassium, calcium, phosphorus, magnesium, zinc, copper, and manganese.

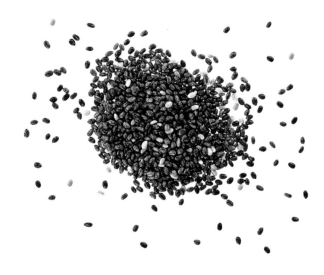

FREQUENTLY ASKED QUESTIONS

Can I wash and chop all the vegetables immediately after purchase, then store them in the refrigerator for a while?
It is better to wash and chop up the vegetables just before you are ready to use them. Hard vegetables, such as carrots, cucumbers, or beetroot, can be washed beforehand, dried thoroughly with a cloth or paper towel, then stored in the refrigerator or vegetable basket. Green leafy vegetables are more delicate; take great care when washing them as they can easily spoil and rot if they are left damp.

As soon as vegetables have been cut, they begin to oxidize. No one knows for certain how many nutrients are lost when this happens, but it is definitely better to leave the vegetables whole until the last moment.

However, if you have no option but to prepare the ingredients in advance in order to make juices an integral part of your everyday routine, then do it!

Once made, the juice will keep in the refrigerator for up to 72 hours.

Can I prepare the juice the evening before?
This is one of the most frequently asked questions, as many of us find ourselves in a race against the clock as soon as the alarm goes off in the morning. Sometimes there is no other choice but to prepare the juice the evening before or even a few days in advance if there is no other way to integrate it into your diet plan. Nevertheless, it is ALWAYS better to drink the juice straight away, otherwise it begins to lose nutrients. If you really do have no other choice, I suggest the following:

1. Use a cold-press juicer as this is better for preserving nutrients.

2. If the juice in question does not contain lemon, add a few drops of lemon juice to help preserve it.

3. Keep the juice chilled and store in a glass or opaque container. Do not pour it out until immediately before use. The glass container can also be wrapped in aluminum foil.

4. Make sure that the container is full to the brim with juice. Making sure that no air is left in the container will reduce oxidization.

When is the best time to drink the juice?

I recommend drinking your green juice first thing in the morning on an empty stomach. This is when your body is most in need of hydration after having been deprived of water for several hours. Your digestive system will also be cleaner and contain fewer barriers, leaving your body free to absorb the maximum amount of nutrients available. Furthermore, drinking the juice in the morning will help you start the day full of energy and optimism. If you cannot manage to drink the juice first thing in the morning, at least drink it when your stomach is empty, as any other food will inhibit the absorption of micronutrients and other healthy substances.

What do I do with the leftover pulp after the juice has been extracted?

Many people dislike the idea of using fruit and vegetables solely for their juice. They feel it is wrong to waste the vegetable solids which are left after juicing. Even if you share this view, it is still not an argument against juicing as the leftover pulp can be put to all kinds of uses. Before discarding it, consider the following options:

1. The pulp can be used to make snacks, soups, hamburgers, or even vegan or raw-food desserts. You can find thousands of recipes on the Internet which suggest lots of different ways of using up the pulp produced after green juicing.

2. Use it as a fertilizer for your plants or in the garden.

Can I freeze green juice?

Yes, but you must freeze it immediately after juicing so that it loses as few nutrients as possible. Frozen juice can be kept for between seven and ten days. Make sure that you leave a small gap between the container lid and the juice, as the juice expands when it is frozen.

Bibliography

Boutenko, Victoria, *Green Smoothie Revolution: The Radical Leap Towards Natural Health*, North Atlantic Books 2009 (and other books)

Calbom, Cherie & John, *Juicing, Fasting, and Detoxing for Life*, Grand Central Life & Style 2014

Carr, Kris: http://kriscarr.com/blog-video/my-green-juice-toolkitvideo-recipe-infographic-faqs/

Cousens, Gabriel, *Rainbow Green Live-Food Cuisine*, North Atlantic Books 2003 (and other books)

Cross, Joe: http://www.rebootwithjoe.com/

Kenny, Matthew, *Culinary Nutrition Program Guidebook*, 2014 (and other books)

Acknowledgements

According to Cuban poet José Martí, "Every man should do three things in life: plant a tree, have a child, and write a book". Little by little I feel a bit more complete each day—and happier about the fact that I am continuing to develop in the things which matter most to me: studying and promoting good health.

It is a great honor and joy for me to present this book as my first small piece of written work. I already had a book in my mind when suddenly an opportunity landed in my lap to write about the very dietary topic which has led to my current lifestyle: green juices.

I would like to thank all the people who have made this possible, starting with Marta Vergés, my co-worker, colleague, raw-food chef, the person with whom I can laugh and cry, my star and my one and all! Thank you! I would also like to thank my family for their support, their time, and the joy we have shared together. I would like to thank Aina Bestard, designer and illustrator, who discovered me through Zahorí de Ideas, as well as her editor, Marta Lorés. My thanks also to Ganesha, always steadfastly by my side. And above all, I would like to thank you and the GREAT little group of people who read my work, write kind things to me, support me every day, and motivate me to continue with this lifelong project.

Namaste!

© Text: Carla Zaplana, 2014 (www.carlazaplana.com)

© Illustrations: Aina Bestard, 2014

© Photography: Shutterstock; except p. 4, Oriol Sánchez

© of the original edition:
Zahorí de Ideas (www. zahorideideas.com)

Original Title:
Zumos verdes. Fuente de energía, belleza y salud
Original ISBN: 978-84-16220-19-9

Design: Mot

English translation rights arranged through Manuela Kerkhoff –
International Licensing Agency, Germany

© for this English edition: h.f.ullmann publishing GmbH

Translation from German: Susan Ghanouni in association with
First Edition Translations Ltd, Cambridge, UK

Front cover: Shutterstock

Back cover: Shutterstock except top left: Ruth Martin

Overall responsibility for production: h.f.ullmann publishing GmbH,
Potsdam, Germany

Printed in Poland, 2016

ISBN 978-3-8480-0937-4

10 9 8 7 6 5 4 3 2 1
X IX VIII VII VI V IV III II I

www.ullmann-publishing.com
newsletter@ullmann-publishing.com
facebook.com/hfullmann
twitter.com/hfullmann_int

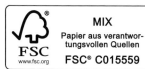